Bikini Body
made easy

613·712

Charmaine Yabsley

First published in Great Britain in 2009
by Collins and Brown
10 Southcombe Street
London W14 0RA

An imprint of Anova Books

British Library Cataloguing in Publication Data.
A catalogue record for this title is available from the
British Library.

ISBN 9781843405306

Front cover image: photographer: Verster Cohen,
model: Nikki Lupton

Picture credits: page 4 Simon Wilkinson
/Stone/Getty Images, page 6 Derek Lomas,
page 22 Mike Kemp/Rubberball Productions/Getty
Images, page 48 Gazimal/Iconica/Getty Images,
page 76 Dennie Cody/ Photographer's Choice/Getty
Images, page 106 Photodisc/Getty Images, page
130 Stefanie Sudek/Stock4B/Getty Images,
page 156 Leo Acker
Illustrator: Maxim Savva

Reproduction by Rival Colour Ltd, UK
Printed by Times Offset , Malaysia

The exercise programmes
in this book are intended for
people in good health — if
you have a medical condition
or are pregnant, or have
any other health concerns,
always consult your doctor
before starting out.

contents

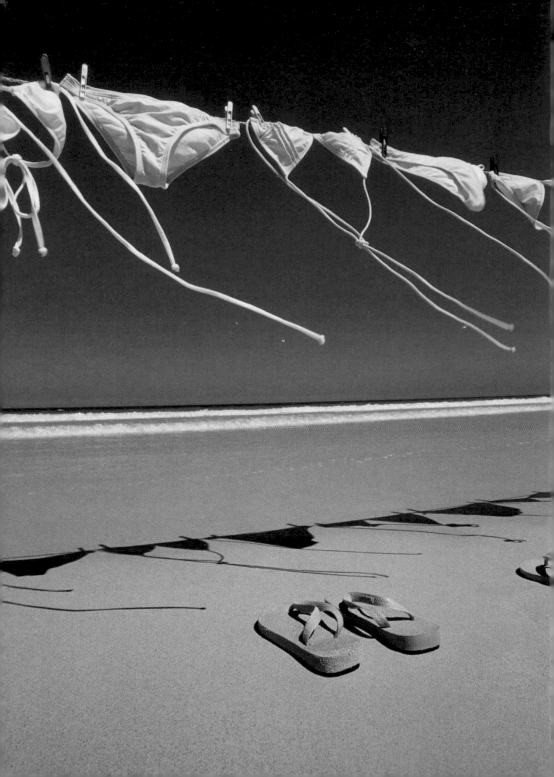

Introduction

Congratulations on taking the first step towards a fitter and healthier you — which you did when you invested in this book! Whatever your shape, whatever your fitness level (and no matter how late you've left it) we have a plan that can transform your body.

In fact, follow our full six-week plan and we can guarantee dramatic results. Whether you're more of an apple or a pear you'll not only find a personalised workout and diet plan to get you looking gorgeous, but also bikinis that will highlight your best bits and camouflage those that you're not so happy with. The workouts are easy-to-follow and the diets are effective but will make sure you are not left feeling famished. We guarantee you will hit the beach feeling and looking confident.

Best of all, stick with the main principles after you return and you have everything you need to be fitter, healthier, firmer and more fabulous for life. So if you have six weeks or just 24 hours, we have a bikini plan for you.

Good luck and have a fantastic holiday!

Mandie Gower
Editor
Zest Magazine

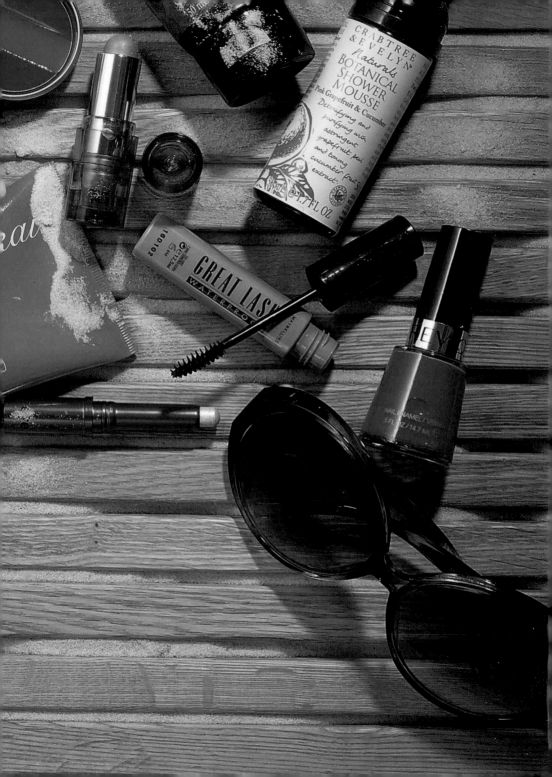

1 **Before** you start

You've booked your flights, you've found a cute, funky hotel overlooking the beach, and your boss has even agreed to let you have the time off. So, you're all set for your holiday – right? Well, what if you've tried on last year's bikini and realised that not only is it last year's style but you also seem to have lost some of your beachside mojo? Well, relax.

Getting **started**

This book is designed to help you get bikini-beach ready in whatever time you have before you jet off. Whether it's one day, one week or six weeks, the eating and workout plans will help you get ready to hit that beach looking fabulous!

How to use this book

Although all women are different, we tend to be one of five basic body shapes. Bikini Body explains how dieting and exercising for your body shape's particular needs is the most effective way to have a body that is bikini fit. This book contains a system of diet plans and workouts for each body shape, so you will find an eating and workout programme that is tailor-made for you. First, read through this chapter to find out what body shape you have, as well as the background to the diet and workout programme, including what you need to get started. The 6-day Detox Plan also appears in this chapter. You will follow this during Week 1, whichever shape you are. Next turn to the chapter for your body shape to find your eating plan and workout. (Recipes used in the diet plans appear at the back of the book). The final chapter gives you some helpful hints on keeping that bikini body all through the holiday.

Your body shape

Everyone naturally has a body type or shape: apple, pear, hourglass, pencil or sporty. Although you can't completely change your body shape, diet and exercise will help to tone your body, and you can make the most of your figure by playing down certain aspects and

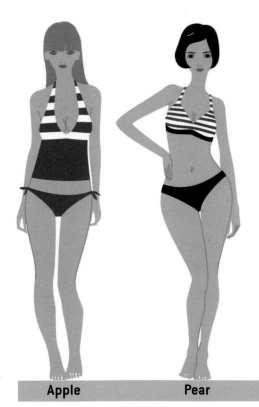

Apple   **Pear**

emphasising others. So, although you can't miraculously change your pear-shape body to a straight-up-and-down ruler, you can reduce the amount of fat that accumulates around your thighs, and you can do specific lower-body exercises to help tone and strengthen your problem areas.

Where the body stores fat

The chapters that follow explain where each body shape tends to store fat, but what factors might cause you to store fat in particular parts of your body? 'There are four major fat storage patterns in women, which determine where your body stores fat,' says Ragdale Hall's personal trainer Dean Hodgkin. 'This is caused by the dominance of the endocrine glands within the body: thyroid, adrenal, pituitary or ovaries.' Each person has one gland that is more dominant than the others. This gland influences the main areas where you store fat. For example, if the adrenal gland is your dominant one, things that stimulate your adrenals (sugar, nicotine, stress, for example) can cause your body to store fat on your back, chest and hips instead of burning it effectively. Other glands and the areas affected are: thyroid (fat stored on the stomach and hips); pituitary (fat stored all over); ovaries (fat stored on the lower body).

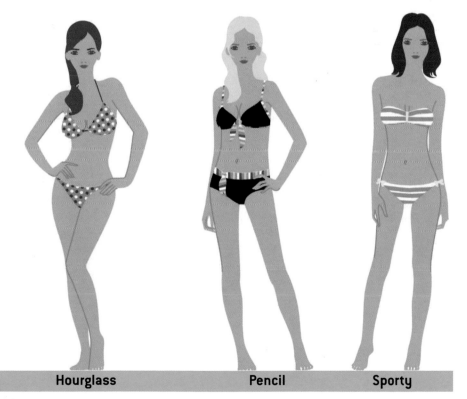

Hourglass   **Pencil**   **Sporty**

Why your body shape might change over the years

You are born with a specific body shape, which is determined by genetics and physical characteristics (for example, you may have your father's height or your mother's thighs). However, you may find that as you get older your body shape changes slightly. 'A pencil body shape will never actually change its skeletal shape, but a sedentary lifestyle and fatty diet will lead to a more pear-shaped figure,' says Dean Hodgkin. On the other hand, an apple shape who follows a low-fat, high-protein diet and exercises regularly will be able to achieve a more svelte, hourglass-like figure. 'Ultimately, it's about being the healthiest you can for your shape.'

What's your body shape?

The quiz below will tell you which body shape you have and how you can make the most of it through the workouts in this book. For each question tick the answer that most correctly describes your body.

1 You have a tendency to stay lean throughout your:
- **a.** Lower body
- **b.** Middle body
- **c.** Upper body
- **d.** Entire body
- **e.** Chest, arms and calves

2 Where do you tend to carry extra weight?
- **a.** Back, chest, arms and stomach
- **b.** Both upper and lower body
- **c.** Hips, thighs and buttocks
- **d.** Stomach and buttocks
- **e.** I don't really have extra weight

3 Which section of your body is toughest to slim down?
- **a.** Upper body
- **b.** Both upper and lower body
- **c.** Lower body
- **d.** It's not that tough
- **e.** When I stop working out, I lose muscle immediately

4 If you could change one part of your body which would it be?
- **a.** Stomach
- **b.** Upper body
- **c.** Upper and lower both need work
- **d.** Lower body: buttocks, inner thighs and hips
- **e.** I'm happy with my body

Results

Mostly As

You're an apple body shape. Apples are generally larger on the top half of their bodies than on the bottom half. They commonly have slim hips and a large chest and stomach. Apples tend to gain weight above the waist or along the lower back, just above the buttocks. This wider waist can make your bottom virtually 'disappear' – making your upper body look as though it's perched on top of your legs. You will want to focus on aerobic training in order to slim down and lose body fat. Work on the lower half of your body to balance out your chest and shoulders. Look to perform exercises that are low resistance and involve low repetitions, such as stairclimbing, walking on an incline, running, squats and lunges.

Mostly Bs

You're an hourglass body shape. Hourglasses are often envied by all of their friends because of their well-proportioned upper and lower bodies, with a distinctively narrow waist. However, if you are an hourglass, you may find that you tend to gain weight all over your body, particularly in your hips and chest area. You should be focusing on cardio and resistance exercises. Cardio will help you to lose weight and keep it off, whereas resistance exercises (such as weights and resistance bands) will help you build muscle tone on your upper and lower body equally. Vary your repetitions and keep your resistance weights light so that you will not build too much muscle mass. Some good activities include slow jogging, cycling (outdoor or stationary), jumping jacks, swimming, bicep curls, shoulder presses, squats.

Mostly Cs

You're a pear body shape. Pears tend to have larger lower bodies and smaller upper bodies. You will find that your hips are slightly wider than your shoulders and that you tend to gain weight below your waist. Pears usually have small chests and flat stomachs. You will want to focus on exercises that will balance out the top half of your body with the bottom half. Use aerobic activities that workout your lower body, and resistance exercises that will build up your upper body. Use light weights and perform high repetitions of exercises. Some good activities include walking, cycling (with low resistance), skipping, leg lifts, lunges, push-ups, shoulder presses.

Mostly Ds

You're a pencil body shape. Pencils tend to be waif-like and slim. You have no large differences between the size of your hips, waist and shoulders. You tend to put on weight on your stomach and backside, although you will maintain your slender arms and legs. You can pick and choose from most exercises. Cardio activities such as running or skipping (anything that raises your heart rate) will help you lose weight in problem areas, such as your buttocks and stomach, but the main focus is to build muscle and toning through resistance exercises. Focus on stretching, sit-ups, fast walking or jogging (alternately is ideal), squats, shoulder presses.

Mostly Es

You're a sporty body shape. You may be a combination of one of the above body shapes, but because you spend a lot of time at the gym, you probably have balanced your measurements out. As well as following your body shape eating plan and workouts, take a look at the hourglass and pencil plans and exercise tips, for extra inspiration.

Do you need to lose weight?

First, throw away your scales. Yes, seriously. Well, not completely seriously, since you'll need them for this exercise. But after you've done this task, then you can throw your scales away. What's more important than your actual weight is whether or not your favourite jeans fit, or whether the bikini that makes you look sophisticated and tanned fits perfectly. Your weight, although indicative of whether you're overweight/underweight according to those weight/height charts, doesn't say much about your individual health. What's more important is to determine your Body Mass Index (BMI).

Now find your favourite pair of jeans, or that dress/bikini, as an incentive to slim down and tone up so that it fits you comfortably. If it's a size smaller than your current size, you'll have no problems pulling up the zip within weeks.

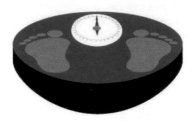

You can work out your BMI with the following formula

BMI = weight in kilograms ÷ height in metres squared

Example: if you weigh 10 stone and are 5ft 6in:
First convert to metric: your weight 63.5kg; your height 1.7m
Square your height: $1.7 \times 1.7 = 2.89m$
Divide your weight by your height squared = a BMI of 22

What your results mean:

Below 18.5	Underweight
18.5–24.9	Normal
25–29.9	Overweight
30+	Obese

Ideally, your BMI should be between 18.5 and 24.9. If it's higher or lower, then visit your health professional to ensure you are medically fit to begin this programme and to rule out any health problems before you start.

Track your changing shape

Taking your measurements is an excellent way to keep track of your changing shape as you get fit. When you burn fat and increase your muscle mass, you may weigh a little more, even though your body is getting tighter and smaller. Here's how you take ten different body measurements — remember to keep your muscles relaxed while you're measuring.

Your measurements might seem discouraging when you start a diet plan, but once you begin to see results, the feeling of accomplishment is wonderful. Even if you have been on a programme for a while, it's not too late — it's great to watch your body continue to change. So, get your tape measure and get started measuring accurately now!

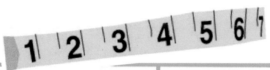

Bust Measure around your bust and your back along your nipple line.	**Thighs** Measure around the biggest part.
Chest Measure around your chest and back keeping the tape high up under your breasts.	**Knees** Measure just above the knee.
Waist Measure around yourself at the navel line.	**Calves** Measure around the biggest part.
Hips Measure around the biggest part.	**Upper arm** Measure around the biggest part, above your elbows.
Midway Measure midway between the biggest part of your hips and your waist.	**Forearms** Measure around the biggest part, below your elbows.

Diet plans and **workouts**

It's time to get started! Now that you know what your body shape is and what areas you want to concentrate on, it's a simple step to begin your six-week diet and workout plan.

The diets and workouts in this book are designed to help you lose excess weight, as well as creating some serious muscle tone and increasing your fitness levels. But if you don't need to lose weight, follow the recommended diet plan for your body type, but know that you can add a few treats, and even the occasional pudding. You'll find that as the menus are low in carbs you'll lose excess water, and will also have an increased level of energy. Ideally, your carb intake should make up about 40% of your food intake, but instead of eating white bread, pasta and biscuits, load up your plate with healthy carbs, such as vegetables, fruit and wholegrains.

How the diet plans work

There is a diet plan for each body shape, but no matter which body shape you are, you will begin by following the 6-day Detox Plan (see pages 20–21). This detox will help to eliminate toxins and any water retention, and you will probably lose 2–3lb during that first week. Then, for the following five weeks (or however many weeks you have until your holiday), follow the plan specifically designed for your shape. Your weight loss will continue at a straightforward, healthier weight loss of 1–2lb each week.

•••➤ Make sure you follow the five-meals-a-day plan: breakfast, snack, lunch, afternoon snack and dinner. If you crave something sweet after dinner and feel the urge to reach for the biscuit tin, have some frozen grapes, or low-fat natural yogurt sprinkled with a tablespoonful of nuts and seeds.

•••➤ You'll see that each week gives menus for six days only – the seventh day is your 'naughty day', where you can eat pretty much what you like. Researchers have found that dieters who give themselves one day off actually lose more weight and stick more rigidly to their diet. This is mainly because after eating healthily for six days, you don't particularly feel like binging on fat-laden meals. Instead, enjoy your day off. Eat sensibly, but order that pudding if you have been lusting after a sweet treat – or have a chocolate croissant and latte while you read the Sunday papers. And most of all, enjoy!

How the workout plans work

The workouts are designed to tone up your muscles according to the needs of your particular body shape.

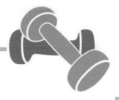

What you'll need
All the workouts use the following pieces of equipment except pear and apple shapes, which do not use a medicine ball.

···▶ **Weights** A hand weight of 2–5kg will be ideal. Just use what you're comfortable with – you can work your way up to a heavier weight.

···▶ **Exercise mat** or thick towel. Many of the moves for your shape will involve you lying on the floor, so make sure you're comfortable.

···▶ **Exercise bands** You can use these instead of, or as well as, free weights.

···▶ **Medicine ball** If you don't have one, try using a thick cushion or a 10kg hand weight to achieve the same results.

···▶ **Swiss ball** (Also known as an exercise ball or Pilates ball.) They are available from sports stores or online.

···▶ **Trainers** Use sports shoes that are intended for cross-training, as you'll be doing some running, power walking and skipping.

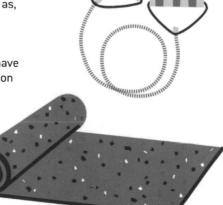

Warm up

Before any workout session it's essential to warm up with some energetic exercise, such as brisk walking, skipping, jogging or swimming. Warming up gets your muscles ready for exercise and avoids injury. Skipping is a great exercise if you're easily bored by walking or jogging. It's fun and cheap and you can do it practically anywhere. Plus, it's the quickest and cheapest way to get fit and is great for toning your arms and legs as well as increasing your coordination.

Your warm-up exercise plan

To prepare your body for its workout, get your blood pumping with 10 minutes of skipping or a brisk walk. If 10 minutes is too much, try 5 minutes and increase by 1 minute intervals each day for the first week. Alternatively, if 10 minutes is too easy for you, try 15 minutes. If you've got some weight to lose, try to do at least 10–15 minutes of an active cardio warm-up every day (with a rest day on the seventh day). If you can, increase this workout to 25–30 minutes each day. Try these:

Skipping Increase your intensity by lifting your feet higher off the ground.
Tips
• Begin with 1 minute, then try to increase by 5 minute intervals.

Swimming: alternate fast front crawl with a medium-paced breaststroke.

Jogging Alternate a 1 minute average speed jog with a 1 minute sprint.
Tips
• Good shoes are vital. Visit a reputable store that will look at your needs. If you're heavier, you may need shoes with extra cushioning.
• By breathing correctly – in through your nose and out through your mouth in a regulated manner – you may be able to run for longer.

Power walking Walk briskly for 1 minute, followed by 1 minute walking extremely fast (almost jogging). Pump your arms to increase your heart rate and breathe steadily.
Tips
• Buy a pair of shoes specifically for walking or running.
• Get to know the correct way to power walk: you shouldn't be able to talk easily. Swing your arms vigorously to increase your heart rate.

Interval training

Between your warm-up session and your workout do some interval training as appropriate for your body shape. This might be swimming, sprinting, cycling or fast walking. Interval training works by increasing your heart rate for a short burst of time, which is more effective at burning fat. So you'll jog at a steady pace for 1 minute, followed by an extremely fast sprint for 60 seconds.

Cool down

After exercising it's just as important to cool down as it was to warm up before you began, as the purpose of cooling down is to minimise muscle fatigue and tenderness. If you feel pain in your muscles after exercising, this is usually caused by the production of lactic acid during your workout. Cooling down helps to eliminate this so that your muscles will be less stiff and sore. However, if the pain does continue, see your GP in case you have pulled or strained a muscle.

Your cool-down exercise plan

The cool-down period is similar to the warm-up and should include gentle aerobic exercise as well as stretching:
1 Do 5–10 minutes of low-intensity exercise, such as walking or marching on the spot.
2 Follow with these stretching exercises, which slowly relax the muscles. Perform each stretch slowly and hold the stretch for at least 20 seconds for the full effect:

Neck and shoulders Stand with your feet a little apart and with your knees slightly bent. Bend your head towards the left and right shoulder alternately.

Chest and shoulders Stand with your kees bent slightly, tense your stomach muscles and relax your shoulders. Fold your hands behind your back and pull your shoulder blades towards each other.

Back stretch Lie down flat on the floor. Bend your right leg then stretch it across your body, holding it at the knee. As you do this movement, stretch your left arm straight out beside you on the floor. Hold. Repeat with the other leg.

Hips and thighs Kneel down, then step forward with one foot. Slide your back leg behind you. Stand upright and place both hands on your front knee. Hold. Repeat with the other leg.

Calf muscles Standing up straight with your feet together, step back with your left leg and bend your right knee slightly. Keep your heels on the floor. Support both hands on your right leg. Repeat this exercise with the other leg.

Thighs Standing up straight, tilt your pelvis backwards and hold your back straight. Lift your leg behind you and hold your ankle securely without the heel touching your bottom. Repeat with the other leg.

Get motivated!

If you start with good intentions to lose weight before a holiday, but tend to succumb to a sugary blowout by day three, be realistic about what you can achieve instead of what you want to achieve. For example, it's realistic to expect around 1–2lb weight loss per week by following your body shape's workout and diet plans. So, work out how many weeks you've got before your holiday and stick to the programme! If you've got 12lb to lose, it's quite possible to lose this in just six weeks – and you'll look and feel better even before you've hit the beach!
Here are some more ideas to help keep you going:

1 Write it down

Write down why you want to lose weight and tone up. If your goal is to 'feel confident in my bikini on the beach', then keep this goal in mind. Imagine yourself looking fit, trim and fabulous on the beach, and summon it up whenever you feel your willpower slip.

2 Don't give up

Don't give up – even if you've given in. If you've succumbed to those chocolate biscuits, don't throw the whole bikini plan out the window.

Just start again the next day (and maybe do an extra 5 minutes' walking to burn them off).

3 Keep a food diary

By writing down every bite you have you'll realise just how much you may be eating each day without realising. Those crisps you mindlessly pick at while bored in the afternoon add on more calories and fat than you might think.

4 Go low carb

Reduce your intake of alcohol, wheat (including bread, pastries, biscuits and pasta), potatoes and sugar.

5 No mixing

Split your carbs and proteins for most of your meals; that is, eat your meat, fish, egg, cheese and tofu dishes with salad or veggies, not potatoes, pasta or rice. Brown basmati rice or millet is fine to eat with proteins, however.

6 Get focussed

Exercise to focus on problem areas. Lunges and squats are the best things to shape up your legs and bum. Follow your body shape's workout, and if you feel that you need extra work on problem areas, add an extra 5 reps.

Confidence tips

Nothing draws the eye more than a confident person. If you look and feel fantastic, then others will think so too. No matter what your weight, confidence is a one-size-fits-all garment that all women should don before leaving the house.

1 Stand up straight

Nothing makes you look unsure and shy more than slumped shoulders and downcast eyes. Go and stand in front of your mirror. Now pull those shoulders back. Suck your tummy in. Tuck your bottom under. Hold that chin up high and smile. See how much more attractive you look?

2 Burn some oil

According to a study in the journal Psychosomatic Medicine, burning lemon balm essential oil can help relax you, and an aura of calm goes a long way to giving off a confident vibe. So if you're feeling a little stressed, try this before you go out.

3 Brighten up

Wearing bright colours will draw others' eyes to you, and certain colours can actually give you the boost that you may need. Try to avoid wearing black and instead wear candy-coloured holiday clothing for a bright, breezy impression.

4 Try something new

If the gym bores you, then burn off calories at a salsa class. Or if you love walking, put on your walking shoes, and take in some walks in your home city — you may discover a hidden gem!

5 Tell everybody else that they're fabulous

Don't wait for others to compliment you. Being the first to admire another person's haircut or outfit means that others will believe you've got confidence to spare.

6 Laugh your weight off

Splitting your sides once a day can do wonders for your waistline — you'll burn around 4½lb of fat a year. You'd have to walk half a mile a day to achieve the same result!

7 Always eat a big breakfast

Think of your body as a car. You wouldn't try to start your car on empty would you? Yet many people run out the door with nothing more than toothpaste for breakfast. Make the time to eat in the morning — your waistline will thank you for it, because you'll eat fewer calories during the rest of the day, and you'll pump up your metabolism too.

Your **6-day Detox** Plan

Each of the body-shape eating plans begins with six days of detox to kick-start the diet and help you feel refreshed. On day 7 of your detox week, rest and eat sensibly. For each day throughout the plan you will eat three meals plus two snacks.

Snacks

- Small pack of raspberries
- 1 small pot low-fat fruit yogurt
- 1 small banana
- 1 slice wholemeal toast with 1 tsp low-fat spread and a scrape of Marmite
- 1 small pot fat-free fruit yogurt and 1 peach
- 2 oatcakes with 2 tbsp cottage cheese and 2 sliced tomatoes
- 1/3 tub (about 100g) reduced-fat hummus and crudités
- 1 wholemeal pitta bread filled with 1 slice lean ham and salad
- 6 tbsp Bran Flakes with skimmed milk

Day 1

Breakfast
250ml warm water with lemon juice (to cleanse and energise your system)
Juice 1 stick of celery, 1 carrot
Morning snack
Handful of walnuts
Lunch
Tomato Soup (page 172)
Afternoon snack
Handful of pumpkin seeds and sunflower seeds
Dinner
Fish in Sleeping Bags (page 167)

Day 2

Breakfast
250ml warm water with lemon juice
Juice 1 orange, 1 pear, 1 apple on ice (optional)
Morning snack
2 wheat-free crispbreads with hummus
Lunch
Chicken Salad (page 167)
Afternoon snack
Handful of nuts and raisins
Dinner
Super-sporty Stir-fry (page 171–2)

Day 3

Breakfast
Juice 1 apple, 1 pear, 5mm peeled fresh root ginger
Morning snack
3–4 celery sticks with 1 tbsp hummus as a dip
Lunch
Feta and Roasted Tomato Pasta Salad (page 167)
Afternoon snack
Handful of seeds and nuts
Dinner
Lemon-drizzled Fish (page 168)

Day 4

Breakfast
Blend ¼ grapefruit, ½ kiwi fruit, 1 slice pineapple, ⅓ cup each frozen cranberries and raspberries. Squeeze lime over; serve on ice
Morning snack
½ avocado spread on 2 wheat-free crackers, with lemon juice and black pepper
Lunch
Spinach Salad with Garlic Dressing (page 171)
Afternoon snack 1 small banana
Dinner
Prawn and Vegetable Skewers (page 171)

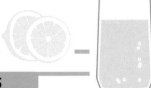

Day 5

Breakfast
Warm water with lemon juice
Blend a handful of berries, juice of 2 oranges, 1 kiwi fruit, 1 tbsp each pumpkin and sunflower seeds
Morning snack
2 rice cakes or wheat-free crackers topped with ½ avocado and tomato
Lunch
Layer 3 ready-cooked turkey slices, tomato, ½ avocado and lettuce for a bread-free sandwich
Afternoon snack
1 apple or pear
Dinner
Broccoli Blowout (page 166)

Day 6

Breakfast
Juice 1 melon, 1 apple, 1 pear; blend with 1 tbsp low-fat yogurt and 1 tbsp seeds
Morning snack
1 small pot low-fat yogurt
Lunch
Minestrone Soup (page 169)
Afternoon snack
Handful of sunflower seeds
Dinner
Marinated Chicken with Prune Salsa (page 169)

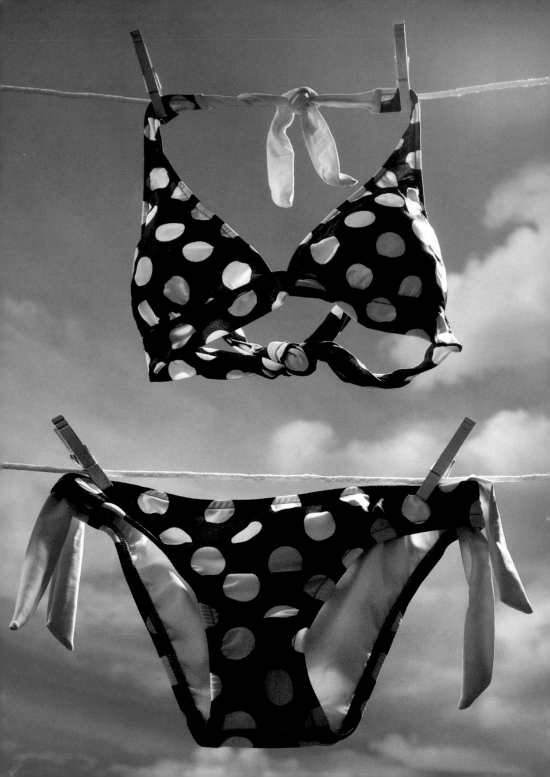

2 **Apple** shape

Over the next six weeks, not only will you learn to love your body shape, but you're also going to find out how best to dress it: both on and off the beach. Once you've finished your six-week diet and exercise plan, your long legs and trimmer figure will create a stir wherever you go.

The **shape**

If you have a tendency to gain weight around your upper body, waist and bottom, but have slender legs, you're likely to be an apple shape.

Your shapely characteristics

The good news is that if you're an apple shape you tend to have long, slender arms and legs, plus a fantastic bust! So you're easy to dress, as you can put your legs on display or wear sleeveless tops to show off your arms.

You have a similar measurement for shoulders, bust, waist and hips

You have a small bottom, which tends to 'disappear' into your legs

You lose weight easily on your arms and legs, but find it difficult to shift it from your midriff.

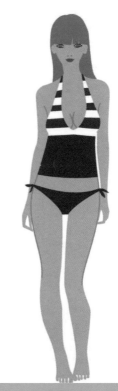

Famous apple shapes:
Elizabeth Hurley
Catherine Zeta-Jones

Best bikini for your shape

Halter necks in bright colours, teamed with dark-coloured bottoms will draw attention to your great bustline and shapely arms, while drawing the eye away from your waist. Since you've got such great legs, short-style bikinis with a belt detail will also give the illusion of a waist. Also, look for bikini bottoms that have a ruching detail around the front to focus the eye away from your waistline. A full piece, with detail around the bust, is also a great way to look super-stylish and toned at the pool. Don't forget to support your bust. As apple shapes usually have a large bust it's important to make the most of your breasts with underwired or structured tops. Shaped tops like these will also give you the illusion of curves, and help to create the appearance of a top and a separate waist. Opt for halter necks, as the thicker straps will help to support your breasts, and the cup size tends to be larger than a bikini cut.

If you don't want to show off your tummy but still want to get a suntan, choose a tankini top that meets your bikini bottom (but roll it up slightly to get a suntan). Choose a tankini with a dark, block-coloured stomach, and brightly coloured cups to show off your best assets, while camouflaging your not-so-good area.

What to wear on holiday

Kaftans are your best friend while on holiday. Team brightly coloured, or jewelled kaftans with a belt to create the illusion of a waist — and use it to hitch the kaftan a little higher to show off your killer pins. Draw attention to your shapely legs with tightly fitted shorts or cut-offs, teamed with loose-fitting tunic tops or floral prints.

What to camouflage

The intention of the diet and workouts is to help you whittle that waist down, so look at cinching your waist in with on-trend belts and waist-cinching jackets. Smock tops and dresses are also fantastic to hide your waist while making the most of your perfect pins.

Your apple-shape diet plan

Most apple shapes desire to lose weight around their midriff and hips, but unfortunately you won't be able to achieve weight loss in one area only. However, the diet is intended to eliminate any bloating, which can make you appear larger than you really are. Although no diet will make you lose weight from one specific area only, by concentrating on reducing the amount of fat you are carrying all over, this diet will help to eliminate fat that is around your waist, bust, back and hips. Eat fibre-rich foods, and reduce the servings of sugar, fat and white carbs for long-lasting and healthy results.

Health alert!

If your waist measures more than 34in, you should speak to your GP about a longer-term weight-loss programme. Apple shapes tend to put on weight very easily around their waist, and this makes them a prime target for heart disease, diabetes or breast cancer. You're also more likely to have problems with anxiety and depression, as well as menstrual irregularities and fertility problems.

Week-by-week
diet plan

The apple body shape is probably the easiest body shape to shift weight from and, because your legs are slender and shapely, your weight loss will be more apparent as it melts away from your waist and breasts. The main dietary angle for apple body shapes is to reduce the amount of fat, particularly around your tummy, so avoid white carbs, but also be personally aware of any foods that might cause you to bloat.

WEEK 1

The 6-day Detox Plan on pages 20–21, which you will follow this first week, is a great body-shaper for your type, and can be repeated on its own whenever you need a boost or to drop a few pounds. Because it's designed to reduce water retention, you should notice a flatter tummy and more defined waist in just a few days.

Foods to enjoy:
- Peppers • Parsnips • Celery • Mushrooms • Carrots
- Pears • Dates (no more than 5) • Papaya • Kiwi fruit

Foods to avoid:
- Pasta • White rice • Bread • Watermelon
- Sugary snacks • Caffeine

WEEK 2

This diet filled with quick, easy-to-follow and healthy meals that won't leave you scrounging for cookies at 4.00 pm. Remember to drink at least 2 litres of still water and to do at least 30 minutes of the fitness workout for your shape each day.

	BREAKFAST	LUNCH	DINNER
DAY 1	½ cup rolled oats with skimmed milk, low-fat yogurt, a little honey and 1 tbsp seeds (try pumpkin, sunflower, flax and walnuts)	40g wholemeal pasta with sauce made with onion and canned tomatoes, plus diced mushrooms and courgettes	1 small salmon fillet, grilled, with steamed vegetables, plus 45g brown basmati rice
DAY 2	Wholegrain cereal (Bran Flakes, Weetabix, unsweetened muesli) with a handful of berries	Medium baked potato topped with 2 tbsp canned kidney beans in chilli sauce mixed with 2 tbsp sweetcorn	Risotto made with brown basmati rice, 50g prawns, plus courgettes, peas and sliced mushrooms
DAY 3	Nutty Fruit Shake (page 170)	Large green salad (try rocket or herb) with 1 tbsp pine nuts, tomatoes, sliced mushrooms, ½ avocado, lemon juice dressing	2 large sardines, grilled, with ½ sweet potato, broccoli and green beans
DAY 4	½ mango, chopped, with 150g low-fat plain yogurt. Add seeds and berries as desired	Chopped pepper, carrot and cucumber salad. Add 75g reduced-fat hummus and 2 slices of wholegrain bread	1 small chicken breast marinated in soy sauce, stir-fried with vegetables and ½ tbsp sesame seeds
DAY 5	Juice 1 apple, 1 pear, 1 kiwi fruit	Mixed salad leaves with celery, sultanas, 1 tbsp pine nuts and a can of tuna in sunflower oil, plus 1 slice wholemeal or soda bread	Kebabs made with ½ pack tofu and vegetables (aubergines, mushrooms, tomatoes and onions)
DAY 6	½ cup rolled oats made into porridge with a little milk. Serve with a little honey and berries	Miso soup (from a pack), brown basmati rice with steamed vegetables. Plus 1 pot low-fat yogurt	Grilled tuna steak with broccoli, mashed sweet potato and green beans

WEIGHTS ARE FOR UNCOOKED PASTA AND RICE

WEEK 3

Your clothes should be feeling looser, and your skin glowing. Use the Exfoliant Scrub on page 46 to massage into your thighs to help break up any fatty deposits.

	BREAKFAST	LUNCH	DINNER
DAY 1	Juice ½ grapefruit, ½ melon, 1 pear, 1 apple	Three-bean Salad (page 172)	1 sole fillet, poached in light stock, with 1 medium potato (without skin), spinach and carrots
DAY 2	2 eggs scrambled with a little milk on 1 slice toasted rye bread	Soup made with stock, ¼ cubed pumpkin, 1 chopped potato, 1 chopped onion, 2 carrots. Serve with 1 wheat-free roll or low-fat sour cream	½ small turkey breast, grilled, with three-leaf salad, plus cucumber, celery, tomatoes and 1 tbsp seeds
DAY 3	Blend 1 small pot low-fat yogurt, 1 banana, 1 tsp honey, 1 tbsp mixed pumpkin and sunflower seeds	Soup made with stock, 1 chopped leek, 1 chopped potato and 5 sliced mushrooms. Serve with 1 slice toasted wheat-free or rye bread	Risotto made with brown basmati rice mixed with 1 chicken breast, grilled and sliced, and 4–5 steamed asparagus spears
DAY 4	Iron-rich cereal, such as Weetabix, with banana and berries	Soup made with stock, 250g spinach (fresh or frozen), pinch grated nutmeg, 1 carrot and 1 potato	1 small tuna steak, grilled, with ½ sweet potato, steamed carrots and green beans or broccoli
DAY 5	Boiled egg with toasted rye bread soldiers	1 small chicken breast, grilled, with salad	Medium baked potato topped with cucumber, tomato, a little feta cheese and pitted black olives
DAY 6	150g baked beans on 1 slice of wholemeal bread (no butter)	Salad of 2 slices smoked salmon, 50g prawns, salad leaves, onion and red pepper, Dijon and lemon dressing	Marinated Chicken with Prune Salsa (page 169)

WEIGHTS ARE FOR UNCOOKED PASTA AND RICE

WEEK 4

Halfway there! Your upper body will definitely be looking more streamlined and toned, and your hips and thighs should be feeling firm and fabulous.

	BREAKFAST	LUNCH	DINNER
DAY 1	150g unsweetened muesli with low-fat yogurt, semi-skimmed milk, berries, flaxseeds and sunflower seeds	Thai prawn soup made with stock, 1 cup shiitake mushrooms, baby corn, pak choi, mangetouts, spring onions and 7 prawns	Salad of 10 pieces soaked and sliced wakame seaweed, 45g brown basmati rice, soya beans, cucumber, carrot, mangetouts, sesame seeds
DAY 2	Juice ½ grapefruit, 100g celery, 100g fennel	Carrot and Coriander Soup (page 166)	Wholewheat or wheat-free lasagne made with onions, carrots, mushrooms, courgettes, canned chopped tomatoes, and a low-fat or dairy-free cheese sauce
DAY 3	Juice 100g tomatoes, 200g cabbage, 1 celery stick, handful of parsley	Pumpkin soup (see lunch Week 3, Day 2)	6–7 roasted asparagus spears with 2 slices smoked salmon, 45g basmati rice and a salad of rocket and spinach
DAY 4	1 egg, poached, on a grilled Portobello mushroom and 1 large sliced tomato	Three-bean Salad (page 172)	Purple-sprouting broccoli and oyster mushrooms in ginger broth, with 20g pumpkin and ½ sweet potato, plus low-fat sour cream or crème fraîche
DAY 5	Juice 1 celery stick, 2 carrots, 1 orange, 1 pear, 1 apple	Medium baked potato with 150g baked beans	1 small chicken breast, stir-fried with vegetables and 1 tbsp cashew nuts, plus 45g brown basmati rice
DAY 6	½ cup rolled oats with low-fat yogurt, a little honey, berries and 1 tbsp seeds	2 slices smoked salmon with a salad of rocket, tomatoes, capers and spring onions	Roasted cubes of vegetables such as peppers, garlic, onions, sweet potato, courgette and mushrooms

WEIGHTS ARE FOR UNCOOKED PASTA AND RICE

29

WEEK 5

If you feel that your lower half hasn't toned up enough, increase your lower workout reps by 5 extra reps each day. Go for it!

	BREAKFAST	LUNCH	DINNER
DAY 1	Juice 125g papaya, 2 oranges, peeled, 125g cucumber	1 small chicken breast, grilled, with a salad of rocket, pomegranate and mango	Stir-fry pak choi, shiitake mushrooms, green beans and 5–6 prawns, plus a small portion of glass noodles
DAY 2	Weetabix with fortified soya or semi-skimmed milk, plus strawberries and banana	Soup made with cubes of butternut squash and onion wedges, roasted then liquidised with stock. With toasted rye, soda or wheat-free bread. Plus 1 small tub of low-fat yogurt	Risotto made with brown basmati rice, 50g prawns, and vegetables
DAY 3	Juice 150g sweet potato, 2 small oranges, 150g carrots	Salad of celery, carrot, salad leaves and ½ small turkey breast, grilled	Small piece of monkfish fillet, grilled, with steamed broccoli, green beans, carrots and courgette slices
DAY 4	Boiled egg served with toasted rye or wholemeal bread soldiers	Soup made with stock and mixed vegetables, plus a little cooked chicken	Wheat-free pasta with tomatoes, courgettes and mushrooms
DAY 5	Juice 1 large tomato, ½ pepper (deseeded and cored), ½ papaya (skinned and deseeded)	1 small chicken breast, grilled, with ½ avocado, lettuce and tomato salad with rocket and herb leaves	Soup made with stock, celery, chopped beetroot and onion. Blended and topped with crumbled feta cheese
DAY 6	Fortified cereal, such as Special K, with skimmed milk, berries and banana	Stir-fried vegetables with tuna	Roasted fennel, sweet potato, carrots, garlic, mushrooms and tomato. Serve with wholegrain couscous

WEIGHTS ARE FOR UNCOOKED PASTA AND RICE

WEEK 6

The end is in sight! This time next week you'll be sunning yourself in warmer climes. So don't fail yourself now – stick to the eating plan and increase the number of reps if you like. Just think how wonderful your reward is going to be!

	BREAKFAST	LUNCH	DINNER
DAY 1	Juice 150g pineapple, 150g celery, ½ lemon, 1 pear	Miso soup (from a pack) Salad of soya beans with 45g brown basmti rice	1 small chicken breast, grilled and cut into chunks with steamed mixed vegetables
DAY 2	2-egg omelette with mushrooms and tomatoes	Mix 5–10 cooked small prawns with 30g crab. Add 45g basmati or wild rice, plus a handful of spinach	Wheat-free spaghetti with clams, tomatoes and capers
DAY 3	Juice 2 apples, 3 apricots and 1 peach (stoned)	Soup made with stock, cubed sweet potato, onion, and ⅓ can beans	2 large sardines, grilled, with potato, steamed broccoli and green beans
DAY 4	½ cup rolled oats made into porridge with a little milk, plus 1 tsp honey, 1 tbsp seeds, plus a handful of berries	Small baked potato with crème fraîche and 150g baked beans	Clear soup made with stock, 1 small chicken breast, Thai flavourings, pak choi, shiitake mushrooms, spring onions and tomatoes
DAY 5	Juice 1 celery stick, 1 apple, 1 pear, 1 carrot, 5mm peeled ginger	Sushi with miso soup (from a pack)	Fish in Sleeping Bags (page 167)
DAY 6	Fortified cereal, such as Special K, with skimmed milk and berries	Three-bean Salad (page 172)	Risotto made with brown basmati rice mixed with 1 chicken breast, grilled and sliced, and 4–5 steamed asparagus spears

WEIGHTS ARE FOR UNCOOKED PASTA AND RICE

Your **six-week workout** plan

This plan is based on a six-week programme of high-intensity fat-burning and strengthening moves. You can choose to follow the first four weeks instead, if you've only got one month until you hit the beach, but the best results will be achieved if you can follow the longer programme.

What you'll need

Remember to check the items of equipment you will need for your workout on page 15.

Workout focus

Although you'll do some work on your upper body and legs, to tone and shape them even more, the main focus will be to burn fat to help you gain a defined and more shapely waist. This will involve Pilates-style moves, as you will need to gain core strength and muscle. By activating the transverse abdominis muscles, you'll find that you'll have a much flatter tummy. Avoid too many stomach crunches, as these just build more muscle and make you look bulkier, although you do need to do some.

Upper body

As apple body shapes tend to have large busts, it's vital to ensure you have good posture. Pilates-style exercises are perfect for your shape, as they help to concentrate on building firm stomach muscles, which help you to stand straighter, taller and stronger.

Mid section

You'll be whittling down that waist with loads of stretching, twisting and turning. These moves will help to flatten your tummy and rid you of the excess weight that tends to settle around your middle.

Lower body

Although your legs are one of your best features there's still room for improvement. Lunges, squats and some high-intensity power walking will help to strengthen your legs and make you the envy of everyone on the beach.

Daily Workout Schedule

10 minutes' warm up
(See page 16.)

20 minutes' interval training
Try walking extremely fast for 3 minutes, then slowly for 1; repeat until you've reached your recommended exercising time. You can apply this type of training whether you're walking, running, cycling or swimming — whichever you prefer. Rachel Holmes, a leading personal trainer, suggests working your body as hard as possible for 20 minutes to burn fat. 'You should work your body as hard as you can, so that you're out of breath and sweating,' she says. If you can, do two sets of 20 minutes of cardio: that's 20 minutes of power walking in the morning (perhaps to work), and again in the evening. The table states only one set of cardio, but if you have the time, double this. You'll reach your reward even quicker.

Weights
Each day you'll focus on a different body part: upper body, mid section, lower body. Do the recommended number of reps, but if you're finding it too easy, then increase your number of reps by 5 each week.

Day 7
This is a day of rest — a well-deserved one! If you're feeling tired and sore by Day 4, you can swap these days over, but if you time your lazy day with your 'treat' day you'll definitely feel more relaxed and pampered.

10 minutes' cool down
(See page 17.)

DAY 1
10 minutes' warm up
20 minutes' interval training
Upper-body workout
10 minutes' cool down

DAY 2
10 minutes' warm up
20 minutes' interval training
Mid-section workout
10 minutes' cool down

DAY 3
10 minutes' warm up
20 minutes' interval training
Lower-body workout
10 minutes' cool down

DAY 4
10 minutes' warm up
20 minutes' interval training
Upper-body workout
10 minutes' cool down

DAY 5
10 minutes' warm up
20 minutes' interval training
Mid-section workout
10 minutes' cool down

DAY 6
10 minutes' warm up
20 minutes' interval training
Lower-body workout
10 minutes' cool down

DAY 7
Rest

33

workout 1

The powerful
upper-body workout

As an apple body shape you probably have great, shapely arms, but will need to tone up your chest area. This workout will help to firm up your upper body, and make those shapely arms even sexier. Add an extra 5 reps each week to banish any 'bingo wings'.

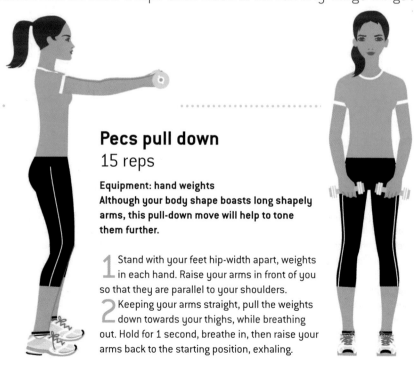

Pecs pull down
15 reps

Equipment: hand weights
Although your body shape boasts long shapely arms, this pull-down move will help to tone them further.

1 Stand with your feet hip-width apart, weights in each hand. Raise your arms in front of you so that they are parallel to your shoulders.

2 Keeping your arms straight, pull the weights down towards your thighs, while breathing out. Hold for 1 second, breathe in, then raise your arms back to the starting position, exhaling.

34

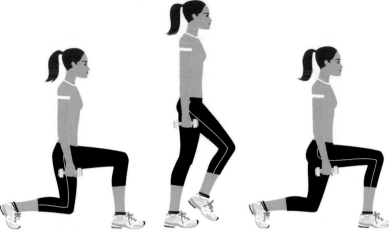

Walk of fame
25 lunges

Equipment: hand weights
This exercise focuses on your stomach muscles and perfects your posture.

1 Holding weights, stand with your feet hip-width apart and your knees slightly bent. Make sure your knees aren't bent over your feet.

2 Step forward one step (a larger stride than you would usually take) and lower your back knee into a lunge position. Keep your arms loose at your sides, with your head relaxed and shoulders soft.

3 Lift your body upwards and lunge forward with the other leg, repeating the above movement. Your back leg should be bent 90°. Your front knee shouldn't be bent any further than your toes.

Super-lunges
25 reps each leg

Equipment: hand weights
This tones your upper arms and shoulders. Pump your arms as you step for a bicep workout.

1 Stand with your arms by your side, holding the hand weights so that the ends face forwards.

2 Step forward with your left leg, about one large step from the back foot. Bend your knee slightly, but make sure it doesn't bend any further than your toes. Now, lower your body downwards slowly, exhaling as you do so. Quickly bring your leg back to the starting position.

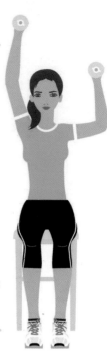

Single arm raises
20 reps each arm

Equipment: hand weights and a chair
This will help strengthen your arms, and, as you perform this seated, it will also encourage good posture.

1 Sit on a chair, with your feet flat on the ground, hip-width apart. Your back should be flat against the back of the chair. Hold a weight in each hand and raise your arms so that they're bent at 90° at shoulder level. (In the 'stick 'em up' position!)

2 Keeping your arms steady, raise your left arm towards the ceiling. Take your time, counting 1 second on the way up, and 1 second on the way down.

3 Repeat with the opposite arm. Remember to keep your arms still and don't lock your arm when it's in the raised position.

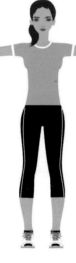

Lat raises
15 reps

Equipment: hand weights
This strengthens your upper body, tones your bust area and balances out the muscle tone between shoulders and waist.

1 Stand with your feet hip-width apart, knees slightly bent. Arms by your sides, holding the weights with palms facing inwards. Pull your stomach muscles in tight (make sure you can still breathe easily and your shoulders aren't tense).

2 Slowly raise your arms away from your sides, keeping your elbows slightly bent, until your hands are at shoulder level. Palms are facing downwards; don't allow your hands to twist. Keep your torso still. Lower your arms slowly.

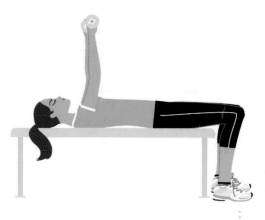

The I-must, I-must bust lifter
25 reps

Equipment: hand weights and Swiss ball or bench
This bust-enhancing move not only helps to firm up the muscles in your chest, but also gives you more defined biceps. Move over Jennifer Aniston!

1 Lie on a Swiss ball or bench with your knees bent, a hand weight in each hand. Raise your arms above your chest, wrists in line with your forearms.

2 Open your arms, lowering them out to the sides as far as is comfortable, then bring them back to the start position. Repeat.

In-reverse pec fly
25 reps

Equipment: Hand weights and Swiss ball
Apple shapes tend to slouch (due to a larger bust and trying to conceal it). This move is perfect for helping you stand up straight.

1 Lie face down on a Swiss ball with a hand weight in each hand, your chest on the ball and your knees on the floor. Your feet should be lifted up to 45° off the floor, but not if it strains your back. Keep your neck in line with your spine.

2 Take your arms out to the sides then, squeezing your shoulder blades together, lift the weights until they are level with your shoulders. Lower and repeat.

workout 2

The **waist-whittler** workout

As an apple shape you'll know that you only have to look at a piece of cake and it suddenly appears on your waist. These moves will help you to strengthen your core stomach muscles and banish those tummy bulges.

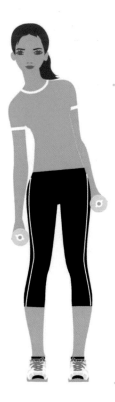

Sideways waist trimmer
20 reps each side

Equipment: hand weights
By strengthening your oblique muscles (the ones on either side of your belly button), you'll strengthen your core, which means you'll have a flatter tummy and more defined waist.

1 Stand with your feet shoulder-width apart, arms loosely at your sides, and weights in each hand.

2 Take a deep breath, pulling in your core stomach muscles and pulling your shoulders slightly back (until you feel a small stretch in your chest muscles). Slowly stretch down your right side, allowing the weight to slide over your outer thigh. Hold for a count of 3, then return to start position.

Let's twist again
15 reps each side

It's an ideal move to eliminate that spare tyre. Keep your legs and hips firm – you only move your waist and upper body.

1 Stand with your feet hip-width apart (your knees should not be locked). Hands on shoulders, with elbows facing outwards. Tilt your pelvis slightly forward.

2 Breathe in. Breathe out, turn to the right, look over your shoulder, and stretch your arms to form a straight line, turning your palms to face the floor. Hold the position for 1 second.

3 Return to the start position and repeat on the left side.

Advanced, 10 reps
In the same position, raise your arms above your head. Link your hands, with palms facing upwards. Stretch your arms to the right, bending from the waist. Turn so that your arms are facing 45° to your body, your head looking down. Pull your stomach in Circle round so that you're facing to the left. Straighten up.

Lateral plank
1 each side for 1 minute

Equipment: exercise mat
Fantastic for targeting 'love handles' and for core strength.

1 Lie on your side, with your lower arm bent so that your elbow is directly under your waist.

2 Using your core stomach muscles, lift your body upwards, so that only your calf muscle is touching the floor.

3 Hold, then return to the starting position. Raise your outside arm and leg to challenge yourself as you progress. Hold for up to 1 minute each side.

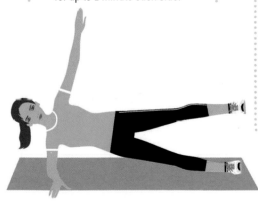

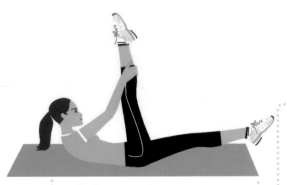

Scissor sisters
15 reps

Equipment: exercise mat
**Banish any sign of pot belly or
'muffin top' with this workout.**

1 Lie on your back on the mat.
Pull your knees towards your
chest. Breathe in, and extend your
legs outwards, pointing your feet
as you do so.

2 Scissor your legs so that they
alternate up and down. Take
care to keep your stomach
muscles pulled in tight.

Upper crunch
up to 10 reps

Equipment: exercise mat
**This one is tough, so take it slowly
during the first week, otherwise
your tummy will be too tender to do
any other exercises.**

1 Lie on your back on the floor.
Pull in your tummy muscles,
breathe in, and on the out breath roll
up towards your knees so that
you're in a halfway sitting position.
Raise your arms upwards, as though
you're climbing a rope.

2 Staying in this position,
continue to alternate your arms
as though you're pulling yourself
upwards.

3 Continue until you've completed
as many of the reps as possible.

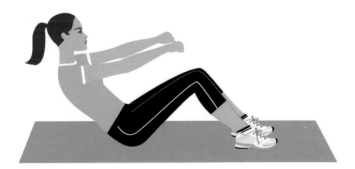

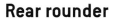

workout 3

The **lovely legs** workout

Apple shapes are blessed with sexy, shapely legs — you're the envy of all other body shapes! Make the most of them with these simple, but effective moves.

Thigh master
25 reps

Equipment: Swiss ball or chair, and rolled-up towel or cushion
Slim your thighs with this powerful move that's easy to do.

1 Sit on an Swiss ball or chair, feet flat on the floor, with the towel or cushion between your legs. Arms folded at bust level.

2 Breathe in, pulling your belly button back towards your spine, and then squeeze your knees together slowly to the count of 6. Release.

Rear rounder
15 reps

Equipment: hand weights
Firm up your bum, thighs and calf muscles with this easy-to-do squat. You can increase the effectiveness by using heavier hand weights.

1 Stand with your feet hip-width apart, holding hand weights with your palms facing inwards.

2 Pull in your tummy as you breathe in. Still breathing in, lower your bottom backwards and downwards, as though you are sitting down.

3 Keep lowering yourself, but make sure your knees aren't further forward than your feet. When your thighs are parallel to the floor, pause and exhale.

4 Breathe in and return to the starting position.

41

The clencher
20 reps

Equipment: exercise mat
Streamline those legs and raise your butt
with this fantastic toning move.

1 Lie on your back on an exercise mat with your knees bent and your arms at
your sides.

2 Breathe in, and, as you exhale, raise your pelvis towards the ceiling to around 45º to
the floor. Pause, then clench your bottom muscles for a count of 2. Relax your muscles
then return to the start position.

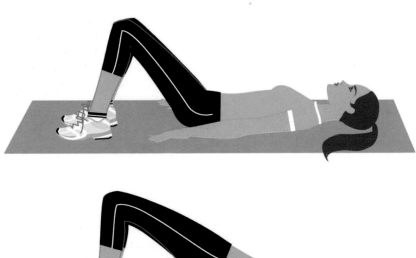

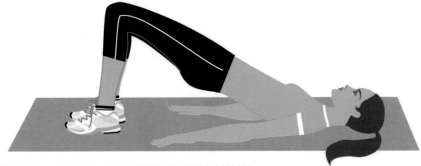

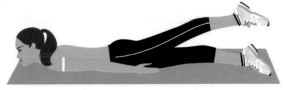

Perfect pins
15 reps

Equipment: Exercise mat
These moves tone your legs and you'll also be working your core stomach muscles.

1 Lie face down on the mat, with you hands by your sides.

2 Bend your left leg slightly, flexing your toes against the mat, so that the sole of your foot is facing backwards.

3 Raise the right leg by stretching it backwards. Point your toes to achieve a maximum stretch. Swap legs and repeat.

Circle, 15 reps

1 From the same starting position, raise your left leg straight behind you, pointing your toe.

2 Circle your foot clockwise, making sure to keep your hips steady and your stomach muscles pulled in. Circle your foot anti-clockwise for 15 reps, then repeat the move on the other leg.

Stretches
8 reps

Equipment: exercise mat
Elongate your body and perfect your posture with this all-over stretch.

1 From the same starting position, stretch your arms forwards, and move your feet about hip-width apart. Pull your tummy in, so that there is about a hand-width space between your stomach and the mat.

2 Stretch your right arm forwards, while stretching your right foot backwards. This should lift your body up slightly from the ground. Hold for the count of 3, then repeat on the opposite side.

Advanced
Repeat with both arms stretched forwards and off the ground simultaneously with your legs stretched backwards.

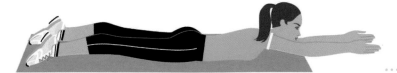

24-Hour emergency plan

If you've only got one day until you're beachside, here's the emergency bikini plan for you, so get going – the clock's ticking!

7.00 pm

Book yourself in for a body wrap, which can miraculously reduce bloating and reduce your overall body measurements by 20in.

9.00 pm

Eat a light, cleansing dinner. Make a filling salad of avocado, grapes, chopped apple, pumpkin seeds, peppers, carrots and leafy greens. Add some non-bloating grains, such as quinoa or millet. Chew your food thoroughly, as this will prevent a sticky-out tummy.

10.00 pm

Run yourself a detoxifying bath, by adding one cup of Epsom salts and 10 drops of juniper berry oil. Relax in the warm water for about 20 minutes. This mixture will help to disperse any excess water in your tummy or thighs.

11.00 pm

It's off to bed, but tonight try to sleep on your left side. This position aids digestion and prevents reflux and a bloated belly.

7.00 am

Drink a cup of hot water with lemon juice. It will stimulate your gall bladder and keep you regular.

7.15 am

Body brush to get your circulation going. Start at the soles of your feet, up your legs, over your thighs, buttocks, hips and torso, then up your arms and towards your shoulders. Avoid your face, but brush the back of your neck.

8.00 am

Get those trainers on! Walk to the corner shop (the long way) to collect the paper and milk. When you get back, do some stretches, squats and leg lifts, while the kettle is boiling. Eat muesli and berries, which prevent a build-up of gas.

9.00 am

Sip lukewarm water throughout the day. A well-hydrated belly is a flat one.

11.00 am

Drink dandelion or nettle tea. These are diuretics, which help to get rid of excess fluid and curb hunger pains.

12.00 pm

Have a cup of green tea: the antioxidants in green tea help you burn more calories.

1.00 pm

Walk to a salad bar at least 15 minutes away and order a chicken salad with boiled potatoes. Wait at least an hour after eating before drinking more water, otherwise you'll just bloat up.

2.00 pm

Mix 1 tbsp grapeseed or olive oil with 10 drops of peppermint oil and rub it over your stomach area in a clockwise direction for what represents 12 o'clock round to 10 o'clock. Then direct the stroke down along your left thigh. (Stroking the left side aids digestion and relieves blockages.)

6.00 pm

Go to a yoga or Pilates class. This will help you relax, as well as reminding you to focus on your core stomach muscles. A strong core equals a flat tummy.

45

Beauty **holiday** plan

Now that you're all lean and mean, it's time to pamper yourself a little. Make the most of your perfect pins with some deep-moisturising cream, and don't forget the finishing touch of a manicure (see pag 155).

Exfoliate

For a top-to-toe all-over exfoliant, try adding sugar to your body wash for a natural, easy scrub. Or try this aromatic blend, which is suitable for most skin types, and you'll also be amazed at how soft and smooth your skin feels afterwards:

Exfoliant Scrub

Combine the following in a bowl: 250g white cane sugar, 250g vegetable glycerine or avocado oil, 2 tsp aloe vera gel, 2 drops lavender oil, 2 drops orange oil. Scoop some of the scrub onto your hand and massage gently onto your skin for 1 minute (the scrub will actually tighten onto your skin like a face mask). Leave on for 3–4 minutes before rinsing. Can be used all over your body.

Moisturise

As an apple shape, if you have been following the bikini workout and diet, you have probably lost inches from your bust, waist and hips. Avoid stretch marks by regularly applying this heavy-duty moisturiser. Use after showering to maintain moisture:

Cocoa Butter Cream

Put the following ingredients into a heatproof bowl: 125g grated cocoa butter, 1 tsp almond oil, 1 tsp light sesame oil, 1 tsp vitamin E oil. Gently heat in the microwave or over a pan of gently simmering water until the cocoa butter is melted. Stir until the oils are well blended. Pour into a clean container and allow the cream to cool completely. You may need to stir the cream one more time after it has cooled. Store in a cool, dry place.

Beauty fact!

Do your teeth bear the truth about your health? If your teeth are discoloured due to red wine, nicotine or just because you haven't made it to the dentist's for a while, then try this quick beauty fix. Rub a strawberry over your teeth, mashing the pulp in. Rinse your mouth with lukewarm water to remove all traces of the berry. Your teeth should now be Hollywood white!

Top ten bikini blitz tips

1 Groom yourself from head to toe. Get your eyelashes tinted, your roots touched up, your bikini line waxed and your fake tan carefully applied.

2 Make an appointment with a personal shopper if you're unsure about choosing a bikini for your shape. They'll give you their honest opinion, plus they'll make suggestions for colours and styles that you may not normally consider.

3 Sip green tea all day – it'll help eliminate any lingering bloat.

4 Try the Lateral Plank yoga move (page 39) and hold for at least 60 seconds. Your tummy will immediately feel firmer.

5 Apply some foot cream to your heels. Your legs are your best asset, so heels on your shoes, or wedges, will show them off to their best effect. Don't let dry, cracked skin on your heels, or a ragged pedicure, let you down.

6 Have a quickie. Sex burns up around 130 calories per half-hour, so go ahead, get saucy!

7 Vow to eat an 'as hot as you can stand it' chilli meal. As chilli is a natural fat burner it will boost your metabolism in no time at all.

8 Apply body oil all over, but especially to your sexy shoulders. If you're feeling anxious, add some lavender and you will feel its calming properties.

9 Choose some sexy accessories to show off your new, firm shape. Strappy sun sandals will accentuate your legs, and a wristful of colourful or ethnic bracelets will draw attention to your long, slender wrists. Create the illusion of a waspish waist with a belt looped through your shorts, or around your kaftan.

10 Hold your head up high. Confidence is the key to bikini success. If you think and feel fabulous, others will think you're fabulous too. So go ahead, strut your stuff!

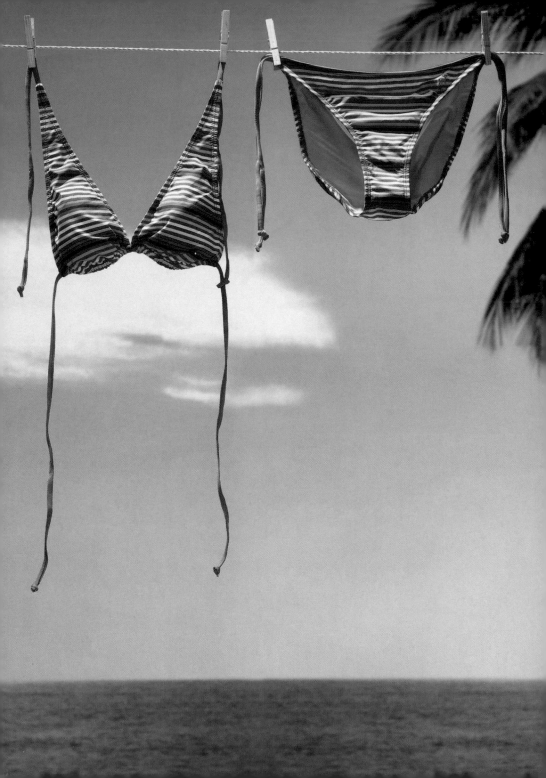

3 **Pear** shape

The majority of British women are a pear shape: shapely womanly hips and thighs, with slender upper bodies. Your six-week bikini diet plan will help to tone up your lower body, while creating muscle definition up top. Follow this alongside your eating plan and you'll turn your pear into a perfect peach.

The **shape**

About two-thirds of women have the pear body shape, and many of them detest their hips and thighs, but this diet and workout plan will turn you into a long-legged lovely in no time at all.

Your shapely characteristics

Like an actual pear, your body is wider at the hips and thighs, with smaller or even petite shoulders and a smaller bust. Even the skinniest of women can have a pear shape (think Kate Moss or Lily Allen). In fact, the pear shape is one of the healthiest shapes to be: women with pear shapes are reportedly less likely to suffer from heart disease, angina and diabetes. However, they are more susceptible to problems like osteoporosis, varicose veins, cellulite and eating disorders. They can also be prone to lower self-esteem due to having a poor body image.

To see whether you are pear-shaped, you need to know your 'hip to waist ratio', measured in metric. Divide your waist measurement by your hip measurement (for example: 92cm ÷ 105cm = 0.8). If the ratio is 0.8 or below, you are pear-shaped.

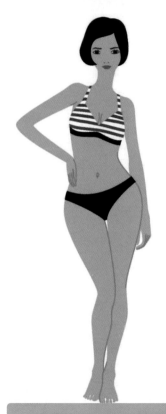

Your hips are wider than your shoulders and bust

Your waist is well defined

You have a shapely, well-rounded bottom

Famous pear shapes:
Jennifer Lopez
Britney Spears

Best bikini for your shape

You've got long, elegant arms, which respond well to upper-body workouts that will create toned and powerful muscles. Your back is also extremely attractive — which is ideal to flaunt as a sexy, erogenous zone. You could opt for full pieces, with detailed, low-cut backs, to show off your best feature. Colourful straps with dark-coloured full pieces will help to create a slimmer silhouette, while drawing the eye to your collarbones and back.

If you want to wear a bikini, you need to make careful swimwear choices so that you can flatter your figure and slim the bottom half while adding some volume to the top. Fight your natural instinct to cover up your widest area with short-style bikini bottoms, as this cut just makes you look larger than you are. Instead, opt for a higher cut on the leg to make your pins look longer and leaner. Mix-and-match your bikinis: a dark-coloured bikini bottom with a bright top will draw the eye to your bust and away from your bottom. Opt for bright jewel shades, with detailed embroidery. Stripes and ruffles on the top are also ideal.

What to wear on holiday

Choose skirts that cinch that waist in: a large waistband will make your waist appear even smaller, or wear wrap skirts to get a more bespoke fit. Avoid pleats, as this extra material will just make your hips and bottom appear wider. For evenings, try hipster trousers in a dark colour to slim your hips and make your torso appear longer. Team with fitted tops in bright colours or unusual patterns. Jewelled or embroidered kaftans can be worn, but they should be slightly shaped to emphasise your waist and be hemmed to just above the knee. Flaunt your sexy shoulders and back with low-cut tops that skim your lower back.

What to camouflage

As long as you opt for tailored skirts and trousers in dark colours, you'll create an illusion of a more evenly balanced shape.

Your pear-shape diet plan

Pear shapes tend to accumulate weight around their hips and thighs and to suffer from cellulite more than any other body shape. Also, many pear-shaped women diet in the belief that they can shift those extra pounds from this area — usually by following starvation-style diets. This yo-yo style of dieting is the worst thing that you can do — as the weight will only return (plus extra!) to the hips and thighs, while your top half remains slender. Instead, reduce the amount of fat on your hips and thighs with a low-fat, low-carb eating plan, with good protein and veg.

Beat the dreaded orange-peel look with these cellulite fighters:

- All berries (goji, strawberries, raspberries, blackcurrants, blueberries)
- Oily fish
- Broccoli
- Seaweed
- Pineapple and papaya
- Organic dark chocolate with 70% cocoa solids (no more than 2 squares per day)
- Eggs
- Mangoes and carrots
- Water

Week-by-week
diet plan

The pear diet plan is designed to eliminate excess water retention and bloating around your hips and thighs. You'll be amazed how minimising carbs and eliminating sugar and salt during the diet will do more for your body shape than all the squats in the world!

WEEK 1

Follow the 6-day Detox Plan on pages 20–21. You should get good results, because it is designed to eliminate excess water retention and bloating around your lower body. As it's high in protein, your body will develop definition and muscles within the first week or so of following the workout plan. Reduce the amount of saturated fat you eat, such as red meat, fried foods and crisps, and add essential fats such as tuna, mackerel and salmon, as well as seeds, such as flaxseeds, sunflower and pumpkin.

Foods to enjoy:
- Buckwheat noodles • Brown basmati rice • Dried fruits
- Lentils • Miso • Quinoa • Rye bread • Beans • Chickpeas
- Tuna, sardines and mackerel • Apples • Carrots • Celery

Foods to avoid:
- Caffeine • White carbs (bread, pasta, potatoes)
- Fatty, fried foods • Sugar • Salt

WEEK 2

You're going to continue with the low-fat, high-protein diet. As pear-shaped bodies tend to suffer from low blood sugar levels, it's vital to eat a large breakfast to fill you up and keep you satisfied for 3−4 hours. Eat one every day!

	BREAKFAST	LUNCH	DINNER
DAY 1	½ cup rolled oats made into porridge with a little milk. Serve with berries	2-egg omelette with spinach, tomato and mushrooms	Thai curry with vegetables, ½ pack tofu and ¼ can low-fat coconut milk. With 45g brown basmati rice
DAY 2	3 tbsp low-fat yogurt with 1 tbsp seeds (pumpkin, flaxseed, hemp, sesame and sunflower seeds)	1 slice toasted rye bread topped with ½ can sardines	1 diced chicken breast stir-fried with vegetables and 45g brown basmati rice
DAY 3	Muesli (page 169)	Miso soup (from a pack) and Three-bean Salad (page 172), plus 1 apple or orange	Grilled, skewered courgette pieces, tomatoes, peppers and 5 large prawns. With 40g wholemeal couscous
DAY 4	Oatcakes with peanut butter	Millet Lunch (page 169)	Chicken and broccoli in mushroom sauce
DAY 5	2 eggs scrambled with a little milk, on 1 slice of toasted wholemeal or rye bread	Three-bean Soup, with a small wholemeal roll	Pepper stuffed with a mixture of onion, garlic and tomatoes, and 100g red lentils cooked in stock
DAY 6	Energy Smoothie (page 167)	Soup made with onion, celery, carrot, stock and ½ can beans or chickpeas	Stuffed Potato Boats (page 171)

WEIGHTS ARE FOR UNCOOKED PASTA AND RICE

WEEK 3

You're almost halfway through your six-week diet plan, so it's a good idea to measure yourself (see page 13) now to see just how much weight loss you've achieved.

	BREAKFAST	LUNCH	DINNER
DAY 1	2 poached eggs on 1 slice toasted rye bread	Soup made with stock, canned tomatoes, onion and basil. With oatcakes or 2 slices toasted rye bread (no butter)	1 chicken breast, diced and stir-fried with sliced courgette and onion. Tossed with wheat-free pasta and ½ tbsp pesto
DAY 2	New You Boot Camp Smoothie (page 170)	4 Ryvita spread with dairy-free cream cheese, 1 slice smoked salmon. Plus 1 small pot low-fat yogurt	50g steamed asparagus spears, plus stir-fried vegetables and 45g brown basmati rice
DAY 3	½ cup rolled oats made into porridge with a little milk, plus 1 tbsp mixed seeds and 2 chopped dried apricots	Salad made with ½ boiled sweet potato, 2 handfuls spinach cooked in 30g butter, 1 tbsp sesame seeds, 1 tbsp olive oil, vinegar, pepper	Noodle Salad with Chilli Lemongrass Dressing (page 170)
DAY 4	Power Plate (page 170)	½ pack tofu cubed and marinated in soy sauce, stir-fried with green vegetables. With 45g brown basmati rice	1 small sole fillet, seasoned and wrapped in foil, then baked. With salad
DAY 5	1 boiled egg with toasted rye bread soldiers	Salad of ½ can butter beans, sliced onion, green pepper, tomato, with lemon juice, mustard and olive oil dressing, plus sesame seeds	Thinly sliced ready-cooked turkey salad (try spinach, rocket and herb leaves)
DAY 6	Blend 1 cup apple juice, handful of blueberries and raspberries, 1 banana, 1 kiwi fruit, ¼ cup mixed seeds	Lime, Tomato and Scallop Salad (page 168)	Marinated chicken with Prune Salsa (page 169)

WEIGHTS ARE FOR UNCOOKED PASTA AND RICE

WEEK 4

You're one month into your bikini diet and you should be feeling much more energetic and seeing some dramatic differences by the end of this week. Keep up the good work!

	BREAKFAST	LUNCH	DINNER
DAY 1	New You Boot Camp Smoothie (page 170)	1 chicken breast, grilled and sliced, in a tortilla wrap with lettuce and ¼ sliced avocado	Roasted cubes of squash, courgette and aubergine, with 40g wholemeal couscous. Pus 75g cooked prawns
DAY 2	2 eggs scrambled with a little milk, with 1 slice smoked salmon on toasted rye bread	Salad made with ½ can black beans, chopped onion, red pepper, herbs and lemon juice	Grilled, skewered cubes of monkfish, courgettes, mushrooms, cherry tomatoes. With ¼ cup brown basmati rice
DAY 3	½ cup rolled oats made into porridge with a little milk. Plus ¼ cup berries	Soup made with stock, onion, ½ sweet potato, 1 leek, fresh rosemary	1 chicken breast, diced and stir-fried with vegetables. With ¼ cup brown or wild rice
DAY 4	Muesli (page 169)	Miso soup (from a pack), plus sushi (try seaweed wraps with soy beans; avoid white rice and use brown instead)	1 small fish fillet (haddock or cod), grilled, plus salsa made with spring onion, celery, ½ mango. With 1 mashed sweet potato
DAY 5	Juice 125g carrots, 250g melon, 1 lime, 5mm peeled ginger, a squeeze of lime	Salad of 75g canned chickpeas, red pepper, tomato, a little olive oil, lemon juice, mustard, coriander, mint and parsley	Fish in Sleeping Bags (page 167)
DAY 6	Juice 125g papaya, 2 peeled oranges, 125g cucumber	Soup made with stock, onion, garlic, thyme, courgette, mushrooms. Blend and serve with 1 tbsp low-fat crème fraîche and toasted rye bread	Stir-fried vegetables, such as baby corn, mangetouts, sliced courgettes, with cashew nuts and wholemeal noodles

WEIGHTS ARE FOR UNCOOKED PASTA AND RICE

WEEK 5

By now you should be feeling great. Your clothes are probably feeling looser on you, and your skin will be glowing. Don't stumble though. Stick to the diet plan — there's not long to go.

	BREAKFAST	LUNCH	DINNER
DAY 1	Muesli (page 169) with goji berries	Miso soup (from a pack) with steamed courgette, green beans, peppers, mushrooms, with lemon juice and seeds	Kebabs of 75g large prawns, courgette pieces, pepper chunks and cherry tomatoes, with 45g wild or basmati rice
DAY 2	½ grapefruit, plus bowl of Bran Flakes with soya skimmed milk and ½ banana	Soup made with stock, onion, mixed vegetables. With 2 slices wholemeal toast spread with low-fat hummus, topped with tomato slices	Wholemeal pasta tossed with sauce made with onion and ½ can chopped tomatoes. With a green salad
DAY 3	Toasted rye or wheat-free bread with low-sugar marmalade spread. Plus bowl of raspberries and low-fat yogurt	2 thin slices ready-cooked turkey in a wholemeal sandwich with cranberry sauce, ¼ avocado and salad leaves. Plus 1 apple or pear	1 chicken breast, baked, with roasted sweet potatoes and green beans
DAY 4	Muesli (page 169) with goji berries, ½ small banana and strawberries	1 large baked potato with ½ can tuna, a little chopped chilli, plus ½ tsp oil	Wholewheat or wheat-free pasta tossed with 3 tbsp steamed sweetcorn, 1 tbsp red pesto. Add ½ chicken breast, grilled and sliced
DAY 5	1 poached egg on 1 slice toasted rye or wholemeal bread. Plus 1 small glass orange juice	1 pitta bread filled with hummus and salad. Plus 1 banana	Bake 1 small piece of cod in foil with 50g prawns, red pepper, spring onion. With 4 steamed asparagus spears, mangetouts and broccoli
DAY 6	Energy Smoothie (page 167). Plus 1 pot low-fat yogurt, with a little honey and seeds to taste	2-egg omelette topped with ham, mushroom and tomato, with salad	1 small chicken breast, grilled and sliced with salad and mango salsa (see dinner, week 4, Day 4)

WEIGHTS ARE FOR UNCOOKED PASTA AND RICE

WEEK 6

The end really is in sight. Hopefully, by now you have lost your cravings for sweet and carby treats. Keep eating three meals a day with two snacks to keep your metabolic rate up and to resist the temptation to open a packet of crisps.

	BREAKFAST	LUNCH	DINNER
DAY 1	Fruit salad with nuts and seeds and low-fat yogurt	Wholemeal pizza base with passata, vegetables, chicken and low-fat mozzarella. With a green salad	40g wholewheat pasta tossed with broccoli, 50g low-fat cream and 75g smoked salmon, sliced
DAY 2	Juice ¼ pineapple, 1 kiwi fruit, 1 pear	Salad made with leaves, tomato, spring onions, 7 prawns and ½ avocado. Plus a piece of fruit	40g wholemeal pasta, cooled, with cucumber, spring onions, mangetouts, cherry tomatoes and 1 salmon fillet, grilled. Plus a piece of fruit
DAY 3	2-egg omelette topped with cherry tomatoes and mushrooms	40g wholemeal or wheat-free pasta, cooled, with 1 apple, ½ onion, 4 cherry tomatoes, 1 small chicken breast, grilled	Vegetable Fajitas (page 172)
DAY 4	Juice 1 apple, 1 pear, 5mm peeled ginger	1 pitta bread with avocado, lettuce, tomato, ready-cooked turkey or chicken slices. Plus 1 small tub low-fat yogurt	Stir-fry 250g vegetables with 50g chicken or prawns. With 45g brown basmati rice or a herb green salad (optional)
DAY 5	Baked beans on 1 slice toasted wholemeal bread	Carrot and Coriander Soup (page 166), plus 2 oatcakes with hummus	1 small salmon fillet, baked in foil, with 1 medium boiled potato and vegetables
DAY 6	Juice 1 celery stick, 2 carrots and 5mm peeled ginger	Pitta bread filled with 1 small can salmon and watercress. Plus a piece of fruit	3 chicken wings tossed in soy sauce and lemon, baked. With a green salad, plus tomatoes, mushrooms and a little feta cheese

WEIGHTS ARE FOR UNCOOKED PASTA AND RICE

Your **six-week workout** plan

The pear-shaped figure usually responds well to toning and strengthening. The key is to avoid muscle-building moves, which will just add bulk. Concentrate on streamlining the lower half of your body — the workout will focus on giving your bottom a bit of a lift.

This plan is based on a six-week, high-intensity routine of fat-burning (for your waist and thighs) and leg-lengthening moves. You can choose to follow the first four weeks if you've only got one month until you hit the beach, but the best results will be achieved if you can follow the longer programme.

What you'll need

Remember to check the items of equipment you will need for your workout on page 15.

Workout focus

Pear-shapes need to concentrate particularly on the lower body; toning and strengthening this area is very important. The workout also accentuates the parts that are already looking good: your upper body.

Upper body

Your best, most toned and slender area is your upper body. The exercises will concentrate on toning and strengthening your arms, chest and back.

Mid section

Your waistline probably needs a little work: a few tummy-toning exercises and fat-burning moves will create some definition in no time. This will involve engaging your 'six-pack' for some proper definition — you'll be able to flaunt your enviable tummy in the sexiest bikini you own!

Lower body

As the lower body will be the main focus of the workout, you'll be doing some strengthening and toning moves to elongate your lovely legs.

Daily Workout Schedule

10 minutes' warm up
(See page 16.)

45 minutes' interval training
Try walking extremely fast for 3 minutes, slowly for 1; repeat until you've reached your recommended exercising time. You can apply this type of training to walking, running, cycling or swimming – whichever you prefer.

Weights
Each day you'll focus on a different body part: upper body, mid section, lower body. Do the recommended number of reps, but if you're finding it too easy, then increase your number of reps by 5 each week.

Day 7
This is a day of rest – a well-deserved one! If you're feeling tired and sore by Day 4, you can swap these days over, but if you time your lazy day with your 'treat' day you'll definitely feel more relaxed and pampered.

10 minutes' cool down
(See page 17.)

DAY 1
10 minutes' warm up
45 minutes' interval training
Upper-body workout
10 minutes' cool down

DAY 2
10 minutes' warm up
45 minutes' interval training
Mid-section workout
10 minutes' cool down

DAY 3
10 minutes' warm up
45 minutes' interval training
Lower-body workout
10 minutes' cool down

DAY 4
10 minutes' warm up
45 minutes' interval training
Upper-body workout
10 minutes' cool down

DAY 5
10 minutes' warm up
45 minutes' interval training
Mid-section workout
10 minutes' cool down

DAY 6
10 minutes' warm up
45 minutes' interval training
Lower-body workout
10 minutes' cool down

DAY 7
Rest

workout 1

The powerful
upper-body workout

Creating a stronger, firmer upper body will give you the illusion of wider shoulders. This will help to balance out your lower body. Don't worry though – you won't turn into a suitcase-carrier.

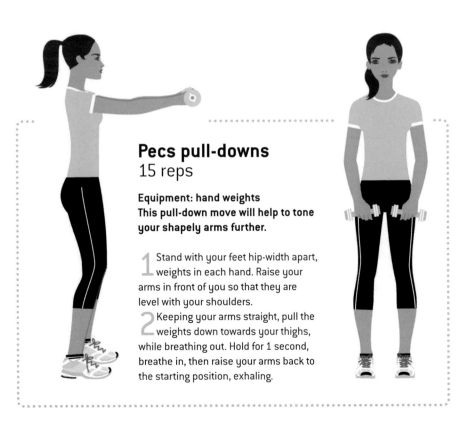

Pecs pull-downs
15 reps

Equipment: hand weights
This pull-down move will help to tone your shapely arms further.

1 Stand with your feet hip-width apart, weights in each hand. Raise your arms in front of you so that they are level with your shoulders.

2 Keeping your arms straight, pull the weights down towards your thighs, while breathing out. Hold for 1 second, breathe in, then raise your arms back to the starting position, exhaling.

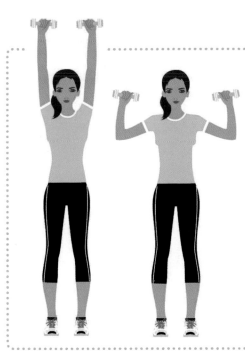

Straight up
15 reps

Equipment: hand weights
Create muscles and tone in your
upper body and banish those
wobbly underarm areas.

1 Stand with your feet shoulder-width apart, weights held loosely in each hand. Raise your arms so that they are straight up in the air – on either side of your ears.

2 Pull the weights down so that they are level to your shoulders. Hold for 1 second, then return to the start position.

Row your boat
20 reps each side

Equipment: chair or bench and free weights
For sleeker, sexier arms in no time at all.

1 Rest your left hand and knee on a bench or chair keeping your right foot on the floor. Hold a weight in your right hand, so that your arm hangs down towards the floor. Keep your back straight and shoulders parallel to the floor.

2 Pull the weight up and towards your chest, keeping your body stable, your back straight and your shoulders relaxed. Keep your arm close to your body. Return to the start position.

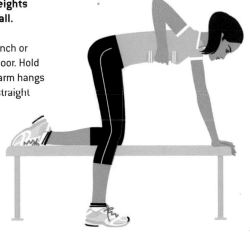

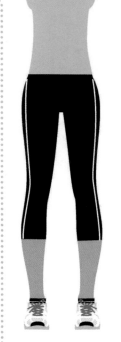

Lat raises
15 reps

Equipment: hand weights
This strengthens your upper body, tones your bust area and balances out the muscle tone between shoulders and waist.

1 Stand with your feet hip-width apart, knees slightly bent. Arms by your sides, holding the weights with palms facing inwards. Pull your stomach muscles in tight (make sure you can still breathe easily and your shoulders aren't tense).

2 Slowly raise your arms away from your sides, keeping your elbows slightly bent, until your hands are at shoulder level. Palms are facing downwards; don't allow your hands to twist. Keep your torso still. Lower your arms slowly.

One-at-a-time lat raises
15 reps each side

Repeat the above move, but this time one arm at a time. First the left arm, then the right.

The big dipper
2–3 sets of 12 reps

Equipment: chair
These are great at working those 'bingo wings' – or muscles at the back of your arms. (If you have any wrist or shoulder problems, you should skip this exercise.)

1 Begin by sitting on a step or a chair with your hands next to your thighs.

2 Breathe in, engaging the stomach muscles as you do so. As you exhale, push down on your arms, moving your bottom forwards over the edge of the chair, and keeping your legs bent. Bend your elbows and lower your body a few inches, keeping your shoulders away from your ears and your elbows parallel to one another. Go no further than 90° to the floor.

3 Push back up to the starting position.

Fitness fact!
Put down that remote! On average we watch around 18 hours of TV a week. But those who have successfully lost weight slouch in front of the TV for less than 10 hours a week. Make the most of your leisure time to feel great and get fit, so as well as working out, go into the great outdoors and get moving!

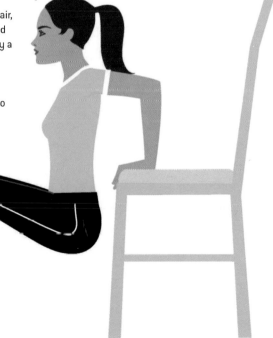

workout 2

The **tummy trimmer** workout

Although your waist doesn't need an intensive workout, it's important to strengthen your tummy muscles. If you find the number of reps quite easy, then you can increase them by 2–5 each week for a greater challenge.

Crunch time
25 reps

Equipment: exercise mat
A flat stomach is achievable with work. Create a strong core with these crunches.

1 Lie on your back on a mat or thick towel, with your knees bent and feet flat on the floor. Place your hands behind your head, keeping your chin tucked into your chest – as though you were holding an orange under your chin.

2 Breathe in, then as you exhale, do a half sit-up, concentrating on your ribs moving towards your pelvis. Keep your stomach pulled in at all times.

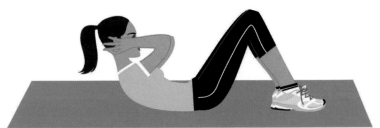

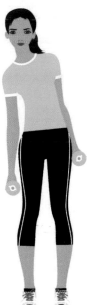

Sideways waist trimmer
25 reps each side

Equipment: hand weights
Strengthening your oblique muscles (the ones on either side of your belly button), means you'll have a flatter tummy and more defined waist.

1 Stand with your feet shoulder-width apart, arms loosely at your sides, and weights in each hand.

2 Take a deep breath, pulling in your core stomach muscles and pulling your shoulders slightly back (until you feel a small stretch in your chest muscles). Slowly stretch down your right side, allowing the weight to slide over your outer thigh. Hold for a count of 3, then return to start position.

The clencher
20 reps

Equipment: exercise mat
Tone your buttocks as well as your midriff with this basic Pilates move.

1 Lie on your back on an exercise mat with your knees bent and your arms at your sides, palms on the floor.

2 Breathe in, and, as you exhale, raise your pelvis towards the ceiling to around 45° to the floor. Pause, then clench your bottom muscles for the count of 2. Relax your muscles then return to the start position.

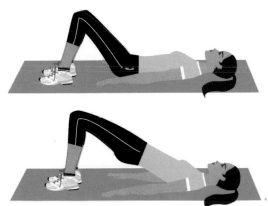

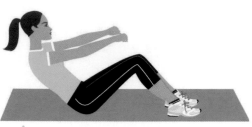

Upper crunch
15 reps

**Equipment: exercise mat
This one is tough but
effective, so take it slowly
during the first week, otherwise
your tummy will be too tender
to do any other exercises.**

1 Lying on your back on the
floor. Pull in your tummy
muscles, breathe in, and on the
out breath roll up towards your
knees so that you're in a halfway
sitting position. Raise your arms
upwards, as though you're
climbing a rope.

2 Staying in this position,
continue to alternate your
arms as though you're pulling
yourself upwards.

3 Continue until you've
completed as many of the
15 reps as possible.

Double up
25 reps

**Equipment: exercise mat
Get those lower stomach
muscles working, but stop if
you experience any lower-back
discomfort.**

1 Lie on a mat with your knees
bent, so that your feet are
close to your bottom, toes pointed
downwards and hands placed
behind your head.

2 Breathe in, tightening your
stomach muscles by pulling
your belly button towards your
spine. As you exhale, crunch your
upper and lower body, pulling your
knees up towards your chest and
your head and upper body towards
your thighs. Inhale, and return to
the starting position.

Back extension
25 reps

Equipment: exercise mat
This move tones and
strengthens your back.

1 Lie face down with your arms either side of your head and legs extended and relaxed. Hold your head up slightly or rest your forehead on the floor. Relax your shoulders into the floor, but keep your abdominals tight.

2 Contract the gluteals and use your lower back muscles to slowly lift your shoulders and chest off the floor. Lower.

Fitness fact!

Another benefit of exercising is that it releases enzymes into your bloodstream, to detoxify your system. Enzymes act as keys that open certain locks in the body. You can think of fat-burning as a locked door that is opened by enzymes.

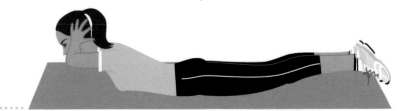

workout 3

The **lovely legs** workout

The pear body shape tends to have shapely legs, but they're the first place that can gain weight. This workout will make sure your legs are lovely by streamlining your muscles and toning the inner and outer thighs.

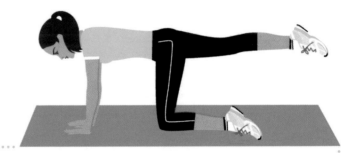

The kicker
20 reps

Equipment: exercise mat
This move really gets those bottom muscles working. Take it easy and if you find that the move causes any lower-back discomfort, stop immediately.

1 On a mat on the floor, get on your hands and knees — creating a square with your body. Breathe in, then as you exhale, quickly kick one of your feet backwards (imagine a horse kicking to be sure you're doing it correctly).

2 When your leg is fully extended, pause for the count of 2 with your bottom cheeks fully flexed. Return to the start and repeat with the opposite leg.

The kickback
15 reps

Equipment: chair
Ideal for toning your bottom and for banishing cellulite.

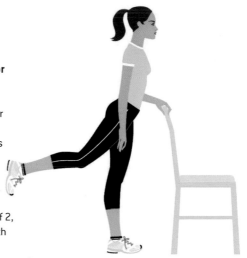

1 Standing with your feet just under shoulder-width apart, breathe in, locking in your core stomach muscles and making sure your shoulders are relaxed, yet pulled back, with your shoulder blades pointing downwards.

2 As you exhale, kick your right leg backwards. Pause for the count of 2, then return to the start and repeat with the other leg.

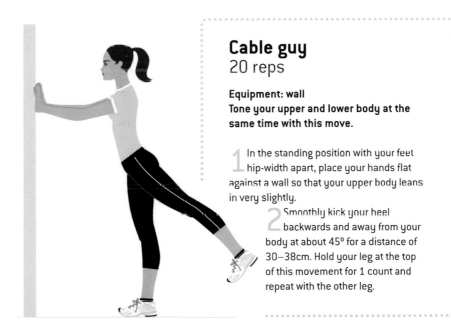

Cable guy
20 reps

Equipment: wall
Tone your upper and lower body at the same time with this move.

1 In the standing position with your feet hip-width apart, place your hands flat against a wall so that your upper body leans in very slightly.

2 Smoothly kick your heel backwards and away from your body at about 45° for a distance of 30–38cm. Hold your leg at the top of this movement for 1 count and repeat with the other leg.

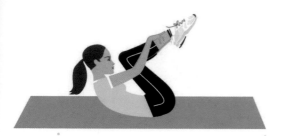

Walk of fame
15 lunges

Equipment: hand weights
Like power walking or jogging, any forward movement will help to build muscle and tone your legs all over.

1 Stand with your feet hip -width apart and your knees slightly bent.

2 Step forward one step (a larger stride than you would usually take) and lower your back knee into a lunge position. Keep your arms loose at your sides, with your head relaxed and shoulders soft.

3 Lift your body upwards and lunge forward with the other leg, repeating the above movement. Your back leg should be bent 90º.

Roll with it
25 raises

Equipment: exercise mat
This massages your spine while helping to tone your thighs and stomach muscles.

1 Lie on your back. Inhale and bend your left knee, squeezing it to your chest with both hands. Curl your head, shoulders and upper body off the mat. Keep your upper body lifted, and bend forwards over your knees.

2 Exhale as you bend your right knee to your chest, holding both legs firmly. Feet together, knees shoulder-width apart, elbows high and wide.

3 Inhale and curl your tailbone to lift your belly up and away from your hips as you roll your spine backwards, vertebra by vertebra. Use a flowing motion until you are balanced between your shoulder blades. Exhale fully as you roll back to the starting position. Keep rolling until you've finished your reps.

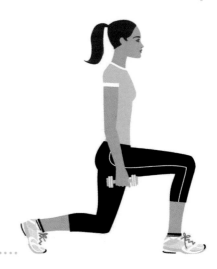

Apples and pears
25 reps each leg

Equipment: exercise mat and step or stairs
Raise your heart rate and get some muscle definition at the same time, by using a step or stair.

1 Facing a step, pull your stomach muscles in as you breathe in, then lift your right leg onto the step. Lightly pump your arms as you do so.

2 Lift your left leg to bring your legs together on the step. Lower your right leg , followed by your left leg.

Advanced

25 reps each leg: Repeat the above, but instead of bringing your left leg onto the step, kick it out behind you, while clenching your buttocks. Keep your upper body steady and straight — don't bend forward over your feet.

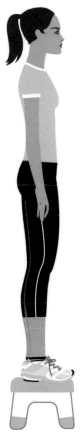
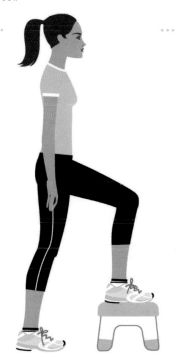

24-Hour
emergency plan

If you've got only one day until you hit that pool lounger in your bikini, it's a good idea to spend a day detoxifying and pampering to leave you looking rested and fabulous!

8.30 am

Kick-start your system with a cup of lemon and hot water. Follow with a poached egg on rye bread and a glass of freshly squeezed orange juice.

9.30 am

Add some grapefruit and lemon essential oils to an oil burner to relax and inspire you. Sit comfortably and allow your mind to relax for 20 minutes. Then, get up slowly and do some stretches.

10.00 am

Body brush for at least 5 minutes, directing the strokes towards your heart. Hop into the shower, wash your hair, face and body. Turn the water to cold just before you emerge to kick-start your mind! Apply a body cream to your dry body. Apply a hot oil or mask to your hair and wrap your hair in a heated towel.

10.20 am

Make yourself a fruit salad or juice. Try a celery, carrot and ginger juice to stimulate your digestive system.

11.00 am

Use an exercise video to do at least 40 minutes of movement. Or do the workout moves in this chapter. Sip fluids often.

12.00 pm

Drink a cup of herbal tea or water. Focus on how you're feeling, but try to remain still and reflective, rather than active.

12.30pm

Time for lunch. Prepare one of the recipes in this book. Sit at the table and enjoy your meal.

1.30 pm

Go for a walk or do some more stretching, concentrating on clearing and focusing your mind. Make yourself a cup of herbal tea, then sit comfortably and sip it slowly.

2.30 pm

It's time for some serious pampering. Cleanse your face with a deep-cleansing product. Apply a face mask, covering your neck and décolletage. Lie down and try to concentrate on your breathing – keeping it calm and even. With each breath, focus on a different part of your body to release tension, working up from your feet to your head.

3.30 pm

Slowly bring yourself back to consciousness. Shake your arms and legs, and sit up. Pour yourself another drink of water.

4.00 pm

Rinse off the face mask, and apply toner and moisturiser to your face, neck and chest. Pamper your hands and feet with a manicure and pedicure (page 155).

5.00 pm

Time for another stretch and a cleansing glass of water, then sit on the sofa and read a magazine before dinner

6.30 pm

Prepare a light, tasty and nutritious salad. Try not to have anything too heavy – fish or chicken is ideal (see Fish in Sleeping Bags, page 167).

7.30 pm

Run yourself a warm bath and add this 'peace of mind' blend: 2 drops neroli and 3 drops melissa essential oils. Immerse yourself fully in the water for 20 minutes before drying yourself. Apply body moisturiser. Add a few drops of lavender oil to your pillow and sheets, and make yourself a cup of chamomile tea.

9.30 pm

It's early, but it's time to hop into bed. Enjoy a restful night's sleep and look forward to a new you tomorrow morning!

Beauty **holiday** plan

The focus for you is to blitz those lumps and bumps! Although cellulite affects even the thinnest of girls, pear shapes are especially vulnerable to it. This cellulite-busting plan works with the diet and workout plan to give you silky-smooth and sexy pins in no time.

Step 1

'Cellulite banishing treatments ARE worth the money, you just have to choose the best one for you,' says Ann Marie Cilmi at London's Bliss Spa. This treatment is massaged into the troubled area to help reduce the existing appearance of 'orange peel' and to help fight the appearance of future dimpling.

Step 2

A daily massage of almond oil with a few drops of grapefruit oil can do wonders for banishing those dimply thighs.

Step 3

Use the stairs as much as you can for exercise. This move will help to tone your buttocks and thin those thighs.

Step 4

Avoid high-fat foods, such as fatty meat, cheese and butter. Sugar depletes collagen in the skin, which makes your thighs appear even more dimply and papery.

Step 5

Avoid alcohol – there'll be plenty of time on holiday to indulge. More than one alcoholic drink a day triggers fluid retention, so save it for the pool bar.

Beauty fact!

Pear shapes may be feeling the effects of all that lower body work, so take some time and give yourself a foot massage. Using an almond oil, add 3 drops of lavender to the mixture. Then, rub your foot firmly, taking time to massage the area between your toes and the balls of your feet. The arch of your foot is supposedly related to your bowel (in refloxology terms), so take care when massaging this area. Finish with your favourite foot cream.

Confidence boosters

Many pear-shaped women have low self-esteem, so life coach Suzie Greaves has devised the following list to help boost your confidence:

⋯➤ If you were an actor acting the part of a confident person, what would you do differently? Write down everything about this person: how they would speak; how they would act; what sort of bikini they would wear. Now act as if you are that person – become that actor playing the part. Be clear about what is and what is not acceptable to you, perhaps – or wear that revealing bikini! Do whatever it is that you feel a confident person would do.

⋯➤ Keep an 'evidence diary' and write down three things you have done differently today that prove you are a confident person. As you build up evidence, so your belief about yourself will change – it usually takes around 100 pieces of evidence before a belief takes hold. Your focus will then begin to change naturally and you will feel more confident.

⋯➤ Make a list of 20 things you have achieved in your life that you are immensely proud of.

⋯➤ Ask a person who loves you to sit down with you and tell you why you are fantastic as you are.

⋯➤ Email your friends and ask them to email you one positive adjective to describe you.

⋯➤ Write a list of your strengths: what are you naturally good at? In which areas do you excel? Now go and do one thing that allows you to show off your strength.

Susan Curtis, director of communications at Neal's Yard Remedies, recommends this rescue remedy to help boost your confidence:

'Olive is very good for rejuvenating low batteries, and crab apple and walnut are useful for regaining contact with yourself if you're feeling low or out of sorts.'

DIRECTIONS FOR USE add 4 drops to a glass of water. Sip at 4-hourly intervals throughout the day. Take more frequently if necessary. Alternatively, put 4 drops under the tongue direct from the dosage bottle every 4 hours.

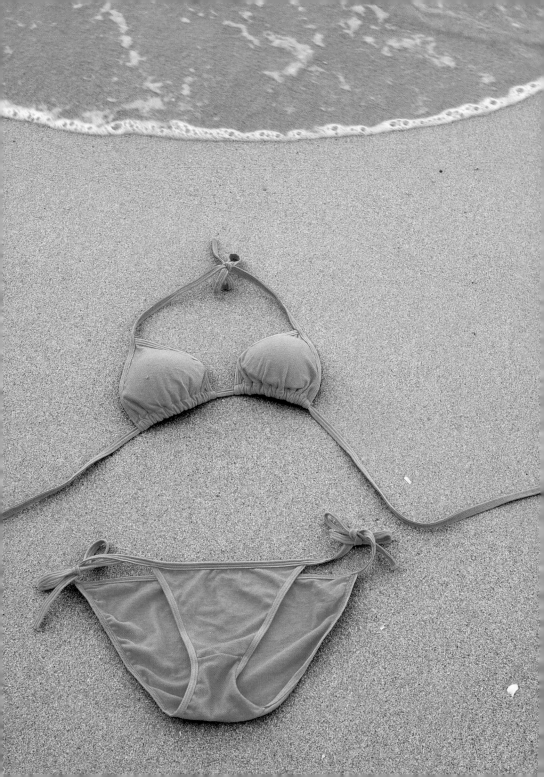

4 **Hourglass** shape

The most womanly of silhouettes with hips to die for and boobs to match. The next six weeks will be all about getting those curves under control and increasing your energy levels with a healthy, low-carb diet. You'll then be ready to knock them dead on the beach with your seriously sexy curves

The **shape**

Think of Marilyn Monroe and you've got the image of the typical hourglass figure: curvy where you want it (the bust and hips) and tiny-waisted, with shapely legs.

Your shapely characteristics

The hourglass figure has long been lauded the sexiest, most desirable body shape of all. However, many women who possess an hourglass figure dislike it, not realising that men actually desire this body shape more than any other as it supposely tells them three important things: first, the woman is not already pregnant; second, a narrow waist shows that she is of reproductive age; and third, she is healthy and free from disease.

Your shoulders and waist are a similar width

Your waist is narrow and well toned

You have curvy, well-shaped calves, with trim ankles

You tend to put weight on the upper arms and the backs of thighs

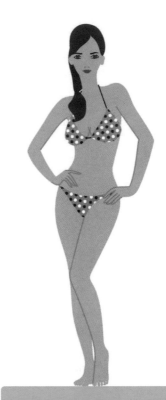

Famous hourglass shapes:
Scarlet Johannsson
Kate Winslet

Best bikini for your shape

As you have an hourglass figure, make the most of your sensual, feminine shape in 1960s-style bikinis with frills, polka dots and psychedelic prints. Plain colours can highlight heavier thighs and upper bodies, so go for as bold a print as you like. Avoid horizontal lines, as these add width; instead go for diagonals or other kinds of prints.

Flaunt your bust with plunging necklines, but make sure there's appropriate support for your breasts — underwired or padded tops are best.

What to wear on holiday

As you know, the hourglass boasts a fabulously tiny waist, with shapely boobs and butt, but what about the rest of your body? You have sensual shoulders that respond well to toning, and shapely legs make up the rest of your Venus shape. Of course, with a tiny waist like yours, you need to concentrate on keeping it flat and firm to accentuate your bust and hips. Choose clothes with tailoring around the waist: flat-fronted pleats are ideal, or tops or jackets with a nipped-in waist to emphasise your curves. Knee-length shorts, with a contrasting belt look good, and strappy tops are flattering for your arms.

What to camouflage

Choose fabrics and cuts that skim rather than tightly hug your bottom and thighs, for a more flattering appearance. If you're unsure whether you want to flaunt your upper arms, then cap sleeves or elbow-length sleeves are ideal. Choose lightweight cotton or linen for the best fit and cut.

Your hourglass-shape diet plan

If you want to lose some weight, avoid fatty meals and pre-packaged dinners, as these are full of fats that will settle on an hourglass shape's upper arms and thighs. But if you don't want to lose weight, but just tone up, then following the diet plan is just a healthier version of how you should be eating all the time. Remember to snack twice a day.

Some statistics

- Strictly's Lisa Snowdon has the 'perfect bottom', research reveals.
- 73% of women and 52% of men hate their bottoms.
- Over half of women desperately wish their bottoms were smaller.
- 49% of women have chosen a small, firm bottom as their ideal shape.
- However, 56% of men are more attracted to women with round, peachy bottoms.

Week-by-week
diet plan

The following diet plan is designed to help eliminate excess weight and water retention, which will not only slim your hips and upper body but will also make your tummy appear even smaller. Try to follow the plan until at least Week 4 for great results.

WEEK 1

Follow the 6-day Detox Plan on page 20–21. You'll undoubtedly lose a few pounds during the week-long detox, but, more importantly, you should feel energised and invigorated, and ready to reach your bikini goal. If you like, you can continue the detox diet for another week and then launch into Week 3 of the diet plan.

Foods to enjoy:
- Broccoli • Asparagus • Mushrooms • Spinach
- Chicory • Melons • Pineapple • Strawberries
- Wild rice • Butter beans • Sesame seeds
- Seafood (although avoid prawns and crab) • Chicken

Foods to avoid:
- Fatty, packaged meals • Sugar • Caffeine
- White carbs (especially bread and biscuits) • Dairy

WEEK 2

After your intensive detox week, you'll find that you're slowly introducing different foods into your diet. But keep up with the good work and you should see results by the end of this week.

	BREAKFAST	LUNCH	DINNER
DAY 1	Power Porridge (page 170)	Minestrone Soup (page 169) with a small wholemeal roll. Plus 1 orange or pear	1 small chicken breast, grilled and sliced. With couscous, and a salad of baby spinach leaves, tomatoes, green beans and mushrooms.
DAY 2	2-egg omelette topped with sliced tomato	Baked potato topped with a small can of baked beans	Small, lean steak, grilled, with mixed salad
DAY 3	Juice 1 apple, 1 pear, 1 kiwi fruit, 1 carrot, 1 celery stick	4 oatcakes with 2 tbsp low-fat soft cheese and salad. Plus 1 pot low-fat yogurt	Small salmon steak marinated in soy sauce, and grilled with 1 tsp sesame seeds. Serve with vegetables.
DAY 4	2 eggs scrambled with a little milk, on 1 slice of rye bread. Plus 1 glass orange juice	1 small box sushi and 1 large tub ready-made fruit salad	Wheat-free lasagne made with chicken and a low-fat or dairy-free cheese sauce.
DAY 5	Juice 1 peeled beetroot, 1 carrot, 1 pear, 5mm peeled ginger	1 chicken breast, grilled and sliced (or use hummus), with salad and dressing (lemon juice, honey, mustard, oil), and 1 wholemeal pitta bread.	Soup made with stock, canned tomatoes, onion and basil (or buy organic tomato soup with basil – such as Covent Garden). With wholewheat croutons or toasted rye bread
DAY 6	Fruit salad with 1 tbsp low-fat crème fraîche or 2 tbsp low-fat yogurt and a drizzle of organic or manuka honey	1 wholemeal pitta bread with ½ × 200g tub tzatziki and crudités. Plus 1 nectarine	Five-spice Chicken Stir-fry (page 168) with 1 layer of noodles

WEIGHTS ARE FOR UNCOOKED PASTA AND RICE

81

WEEK 3

By now your clothes should be looser and your shape more defined. Keep to the diet, avoiding sugary or salty snacks, as these can bloat your tummy and prevent further weight loss.

	BREAKFAST	LUNCH	DINNER
DAY 1	1 boiled egg with toasted rye or wheat-free bread	1 small wholemeal roll filled with 2 tsp low-fat spread, 1 slice lean ham and salad. Plus 1 small pot low-fat yogurt and 1 small banana	Tuna and Sweetcorn Pesto Pasta (page 172) with salad
DAY 2	Grape Shakes (page 168)	Ready-made sandwich, wrap, roll or salad. Choose chicken or tuna, with salad and low-fat cottage cheese or spread	Beef Fajitas (page 166) with 1 tbsp each of guacamole, grated reduced-fat Cheddar and salsa, plus salad. (Use ready-made salsa, or make your own)
DAY 3	2-egg-white omelette topped with tomatoes and mushrooms	1 small box sushi and 1 large tub ready-made fruit salad	1 lean, loin lamb chop, grilled, with 1 sweet potato, mashed, 1 tsp low-fat spread, vegetables and mint sauce
DAY 4	Juice 2 green apples, 1 kiwi fruit, 1 celery stick, 5mm peeled ginger. Plus 1 small slice wholemeal toast with low-fat peanut butter	Large mixed salad, without dressing, with 1 small can tuna or salmon chunks	1 small chicken breast, grilled and sliced, with stir-fried broccoli, green beans and mushrooms. Add a dash of soy sauce and 1 tsp sesame seeds (optional)
DAY 5	1 small banana, 1 kiwi fruit and 1 pot fat-free natural yogurt	2 small slices smoked salmon with salad leaves	Moroccan Lamb (page 169) with 25g couscous or a small baked potato and broccoli
DAY 6	Juice 1 apple, a handful of grapes, 1 orange and 1 nectarine. Plus 1 small tub low-fat yogurt	Bowl of Carrot and Coriander Soup (page 166) or Minestrone Soup (page 169), with 1 small wholemeal roll	Small tuna steak, grilled, with 25g wild rice and steamed mixed vegetables

WEIGHTS ARE FOR UNCOOKED PASTA AND RICE

WEEK 4

Well done! You've done fantastically well, and you should be feeling energised and motivated. If you're getting hungry after your main meal, eat a piece of fruit or a few nuts.

	BREAKFAST	LUNCH	DINNER
DAY 1	2 slices wholemeal toast with 2 tsp each of low-fat spread and honey	Rocket and Parmesan cheese salad, without dressing (add tomato slices and lemon juice if you like). Plus 1 small pot low-fat yogurt	Garlic Mushroom Spaghetti (page 168)
DAY 2	1 wholemeal fruit scone with 2 tsp low-fat spread and a handful of grapes	Cubes of vegetables such as squash, courgette, aubergine tossed in 1 tbsp oil and roasted (or sliced and grilled)	Grilled tuna steak and avocado slices with tomato chunks and feta cheese. Add some roasted pine nuts and a herb salad
DAY 3	6 tbsp Bran Flakes with 1 tbsp raisins, a few raspberries and a little skimmed milk	150g melon or 2 fresh figs with 3 slices Parma ham	Tuna Meatballs (page 172)
DAY 4	3 tbsp unsweetened muesli with a little skimmed milk and 1 apple	Slice 3 tomatoes and 1 pack mozzarella and serve over lettuce leaves. Add lemon juice and black pepper	1 small chicken breast, grilled and served with grilled courgettes and peppers
DAY 5	2 slices wholemeal toast with 2 tsp peanut butter and 1 small banana	Carrot and Coriander Soup (page 166)	1 small fish fillet (haddock or cod), grilled. With salad or steamed vegetables
DAY 6	2 Weetabix with skimmed milk and a few strawberries, plus 1 small glass of fresh orange juice	Miso soup (from a pack) with 1 small box sushi	Fish Pie (page 167) with steamed vegetables

WEIGHTS ARE FOR UNCOOKED PASTA AND RICE

WEEK 5

Not long to go now! You should be feeling and looking fantastic and are probably the envy of your friends and workmates. Buy yourself a treat to reward your good work.

	BREAKFAST	LUNCH	DINNER
DAY 1	2 slices wholemeal toast with 2 tsp each low-fat spread and marmalade, plus 1 nectarine	Ryvita with 4 ready-cooked turkey breast slices, lettuce and tomato, plus low-fat cream cheese (optional).	1 small skinless chicken breast, grilled, with salad or steamed vegetables
DAY 2	1 skinny latte, 1 reduced-sugar cereal bar and 1 small banana	2 slices smoked salmon with herb salad and lemon wedges for dressing	1 small fillet of fish (haddock or cod), grilled, with 30g cherry tomatoes simmered until almost liquid, plus 1 tbsp fresh basil. Serve with 35g wholemeal pasta
DAY 3	Muesli (page 169), plus 1 glass pineapple juice	Slice of roasted lean beef with watercress and 1 tsp horseradish, tomatoes and spring onions, plus 2 Ryvita	Cottage Pie (page 167) with steamed vegetables
DAY 4	Juice ½ pineapple and 1 kiwi fruit	Salad of 1 boiled medium potato, lettuce, tomatoes, onion, a small can of tuna, and 1 hard-boiled egg	Ginger and Garlic Beef (page 168) with 45g brown basmati rice
DAY 5	2 eggs scrambled with a little milk, small slice smoked salmon and low-fat cream cheese on 1 slice toasted rye bread	Minestrone Soup (page 169)	1 chicken breast, grilled, with 4–5 steamed asparagus spears. Cook risotto (from a pack), stir in sliced chicken and asparagus. Add a dash of olive oil and lemon juice
DAY 6	½ cup rolled oats made into porridge with a little milk, plus 1 tsp honey, 1 tbsp mixed seeds	75g feta cheese, cubed and tossed with a salad of lettuce, tomatoes, onion and 6 olives, served with a small roll	Small tuna steak, grilled, with steamed purple-sprouting broccoli and green beans

WEIGHTS ARE FOR UNCOOKED PASTA AND RICE

WEEK 6

This is the final stage. If you've followed the diet and workouts faithfully you'll soon reach your goal, but if you feel that you haven't lost enough weight, swap this week with Week 1's 6-day Detox Plan to help shift the last pounds.

	BREAKFAST	LUNCH	DINNER
DAY 1	Energy Smoothie (page 167)	1 chicken breast, grilled and sliced. Add to 45g brown basmati rice, 1 spring onion, sliced mushrooms, ¼ cup peas and 5 mangetouts	Soup made with stock, ½ chopped onion, 1 medium potato, 1 leek. Serve with wholemeal roll or croutons
DAY 2	1 boiled egg with toasted rye-bread soldiers	4 Ryvita with low-fat cream cheese and 2 smoked salmon slices, plus tomatoes or ½ avocado and lemon juice	Paprika Pork (page 170) with a small jacket potato and steamed broccoli
DAY 3	Muesli (page 169)	50g sliced mozzarella and ½ sliced avocado, with tomato chunks, spring onions and rocket salad	Baked Spicy Chicken and Rice (page 166). Plus fruit, low-fat yogurt and 1 square of dark chocolate, grated
DAY 4	Juice 1 celery stick, 1 carrot, 1 kiwi fruit, 5mm peeled ginger	½ small can of fish (tuna, salmon, mackerel) with tomato and cucumber, and 1 tsp low-fat mayonnaise, plus 2 Ryvita or 4 oatcakes	Vietnamese Chicken Noodle Soup (page 173)
DAY 5	1 egg, poached, on rye or wholemeal toast	½ avocado in chunks, with mixed herbs and salad and 2 tbsp toasted pine nuts	Thai Salmon (page 172) with 3 small, boiled new potatoes and green vegetables
DAY 6	½ cup rolled oats made into porridge with a little milk, plus 1 tsp honey and 1 tbsp mixed seeds	150g ready-cooked sliced turkey breast with ½ sliced avocado, tomato, spring onions, lemon juice dressing	Baked Spicy Chicken and Rice (page 166)

WEIGHTS ARE FOR UNCOOKED PASTA AND RICE

Your **six-week workout** plan

The hourglass figure is an enviable one but it's important to keep those curves in check. The following workout will help to tone and slim your hips and upper arms. If there's a particular area you'd like to focus on, increase the number of reps by 2–5 for each week you follow the workout plan.

What you'll need

Remember to check the items of equipment you will need for your workout on page 15.

Workout focus

The hourglass shape is very lucky: there's virtually no area of this body shape you'd want to hide. However, it's easy for an untoned hourglass shape to gather weight on the hips and thighs. Without regular workouts, the upper body may also collect fat, so arm-strengthening and toning exercises are a must in any exercise plan.

The workout focuses on whittling down that waist even more, to ensure the eye is drawn to your best area. By using strengthening upper body work you will also appear taller, stronger and more powerful, while leg lengthening and toning exercises will ensure your bottom and thighs are curvy, not wobbly. You will also find that your figure particularly benefits from the interval training.

Upper body

The main feature of the upper body in the hourglass figure is your bust. When exercising, make sure you wear a good sports bra, to keep your bust line firm and healthy. Fitness expert Nikki Waterman says, 'Unsupported breasts can bounce up to 14cm during exercise, which leads to breast-health problems later in life.' The Shock Absorber D+ Max sports bra reduces breast bounce by 74%.

Mid section

Although your waist probably needs very little work, as it's usually flat and toned, the workout will make sure that it's strong.

Lower body

A curvaceous bottom should never be underestimated, but the secret is to keep your curves while firming and toning. Otherwise your bottom can 'slump' over your legs, making you look wider than you really are. The workout will lift those cheeks, while elongating your legs for the sexiest shape of all!

Daily Workout Schedule

10 minutes' warm up
(See page 16.)

30 minutes' interval training
The hourglass body shape's goal is to improve your overall fitness, as well as to burn excess fat from your upper body and thighs, without losing those sexy curves. Try interval training in the pool, the park or on your bike. Try sprinting or cycling for 40 seconds, followed by a 2 minute slower jog. In the pool, swim 5 average-speed laps, then 1 lap at 'Olympic' speed. You should be out of breath at the end of each fast section of your training, and unable to carry out a conversation at all times.

Weights
Each day you'll focus on a different body part: upper body, mid section, lower body. Do the recommended number of reps, but If you're finding it too easy, then increase your number of reps by 5 each week.

Day 7
This is a day of rest – a well-deserved one! If you're feeling tired and sore by Day 4, you can swap these days over, but if you time your lazy day with your 'treat' day you'll definitely feel more relaxed and pampered.

10 minutes' cool down
(See page 17.)

DAY 1
10 minutes' warm up
30 minutes' interval training
Upper-body workout
10 minutes' cool down

DAY 2
10 minutes' warm up
30 minutes' interval training
Mid-section workout
10 minutes' cool down

DAY 3
10 minutes' warm up
30 minutes' interval training
Lower-body workout
10 minutes' cool down

DAY 4
10 minutes' warm up
30 minutes' interval training
Upper-body workout
10 minutes' cool down

DAY 5
10 minutes' warm up
30 minutes' interval training
Mid-section workout
10 minutes' cool down

DAY 6
10 minutes' warm up
30 minutes' interval training
Lower-body workout
10 minutes' cool down

DAY 7
Rest

workout 1

The **better breasts** and **shapely shoulders** workout

Hourglass body shapes have great breasts and long, elegant arms. Make the most of your womanly figure by defining your biceps and 'bingo wings', and emphasising your collarbone. You'll look leaner, stronger and even a little bit taller.

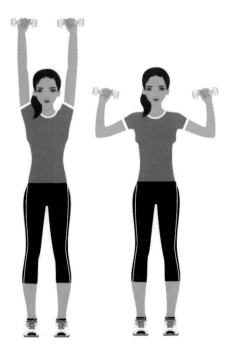

Straight up
30 reps each side

Equipment: hand weights
These moves create muscles and tone in your upper body and banish those wobbly underarm areas.

1 Stand with your feet shoulder-width apart, weights held loosely in each hand. Raise your arms so that they are straight up in the air – on either side of your ears.

2 Pull the weights down so that they are level with your shoulders. Hold for 1 second, then return to the start position.

Push up
30 reps

Equipment: exercise mat
This is an easy version of a push-up, but gives great results.

1 Kneel on an exercise mat in the push-up position. Breathe in, keeping your stomach muscles firm and tight.

2 Lower your body to the mat, making sure your bottom is level with your back and thighs. Hold, then return to start.

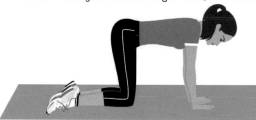

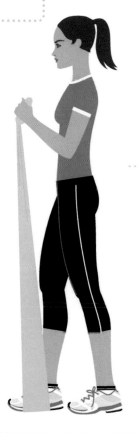

Popeye curl
30 reps
(increase by 10 reps each week)

Equipment: exercise band or hand weights
The fitness band increases your intensity by around 50%. Take it slowly so that you don't pull any muscles.

1 Stand with one foot on the exercise band. Grip the ends of the band with each hand (or hold the free weights). Bend your left arm towards your shoulder, making sure you don't sway, or lean towards the right. Keep your right arm steady against your thigh.

2 Lower your left arm, then repeat with your right arm. Don't rush the move – keep it slow and controlled.

Take a seat
2 × 15 reps

Equipment: exercise band and mat
A simple exercise band emulates a gym-machine workout.

1 Sit on the floor with your knees slightly bent and your back straight. Hold an exercise band around your feet. Your hands should be more or less in line with your knees and your arms shoulder-width apart. Keep your shoulders down and look straight ahead, keeping your shoulders soft.

2 Breathe in, then exhale, pulling the exercise band towards you and squeezing your shoulder blades together. Keep your stomach muscles pulled in to support your posture. Return to the starting position.

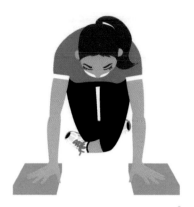

Bookworm
10 reps

Equipment: two fitness blocks or two large books (about 10cm thick)
This is a serious yoga-based move that tones the wrists and arms, as well as strengthening your tummy muscles.

1 Using two blocks, kneel down with your ankles crossed under your bottom. Place the blocks either side of you and put your hands flat on them.

2 Breathe in, press your hands down and try to pull your thighs up towards your upper body, bringing your heels towards your buttocks. Hold for 5 breaths.

Ladder climb
15 steps

Equipment: exercise mat
Works your tummy muscles as well as your inner thighs.

1 Lie on your back, knees bent. Bring your legs straight up, at a right angle to the floor. Make sure your stomach is pressed towards the floor at all times.

2 Bring your right foot down about 30cm. Lower your left foot level to meet your right. Then lower your right foot down another step. Repeat with your left. Now walk your legs back up in steps.

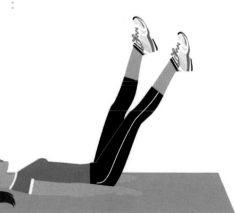

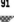

workout 2

The **waspish-waist** workout

Make the most of your waist by ensuring it's flat and toned as well as strong. A powerful core area helps to prevent back pain, and encourages good posture. As hourglass figures tend to have larger bosoms, it's important to keep your shoulders pulled back and your tummy muscles tight, otherwise you'll slouch (and look 5lb heavier).

Let's twist again
7 reps each side

Equipment: exercise mat and block or cushion
Use your thigh muscles to increase the core strength of your waist, as this will need to remain strong and firm.

1 Lie on your back, arms out to the sides. Bend your knees and place a block or cushion between them. Lift so that your shins are parallel to the floor, at right angles to your thighs. Pull in your lower belly.

2 Exhale and lower your knees to just above the floor to the right. Inhale and bring your legs back to the centre by grounding your left side. Repeat the move on the other side.

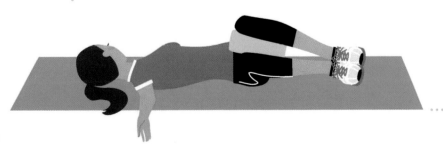

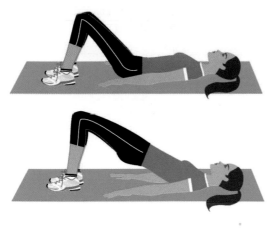

The clencher
5 reps

Equipment: exercise mat
Tone your buttocks as
well as your midriff with this
basic Pilates move.

1 Lie on your back on an exercise mat with your knees bent and your arms at your sides, palms on the floor.

2 Breathe in, and, as you exhale, raise your pelvis towards the ceiling to around 45° to the floor. Pause, then clench your bottom muscles for the count of 2. Relax your muscles then return to the start position.

The kicker
15 reps each side

Equipment: exercise mat
This move really gets those
lower-stomach muscles
working, but stop if you find
any lower back discomfort.

1 Get on your hands and knees – creating a square with your body. Breathe in, then as you exhale, kick one of your feet backwards.

2 When your leg is fully extended, pause for a count of 2 with your bottom cheeks fully flexed. Return to the start and repeat with the opposite leg.

Advanced
Reach the opposite arm forwards and hold for a count of 3.

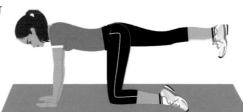

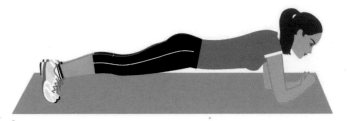

Walk the plank

hold for 30 seconds, increasing to 60 seconds

Equipment: exercise mat
This move may look easy, but it's a real killer! Begin slowly and increase gradually.

1 Position your body so that your toes are on the ground and your elbows are directly below your shoulders. Raise yourself up, keeping a straight line from your shoulders.

2 Use your abdominals to maintain the position. Keep your body straight and don't raise your bottom too high. Hold.

Belle of the ball

20 reps

Equipment: Swiss ball
This will challenge your stomach muscles and thighs.

1 Sit on the Swiss ball, with your feet firmly in front of you, arms behind your head. Take small steps and move your legs forward so that your body begins to move down the ball towards the floor. Once the ball reaches the middle of your back, pause and breathe deeply, tightening your stomach muscles.

2 Inhale, and raise your upper body off the ball (to the middle of your back, just under your bra line). You should feel your stomach muscles tighten. Hold, then lower to the start position, as slowly as possible.

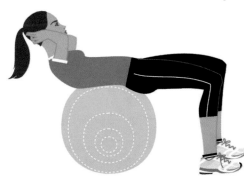

Good medicine
15 reps

Equipment: exercise mat and medicine ball or free weights This is a great move to create definition on either side of your abs.

1 Sit down with your legs bent, feet flat on the floor in front of you. Holding the medicine ball in both hands, rock backwards slightly to engage your stomach muscles as you lift your feet off the floor.

2 Holding the ball out in front of you, elbows slightly bent, rotate your shoulders round and twist from the waist from left to right, feeling your abdominal muscles working at the front and sides of your stomach.
Swivel left and right 15 times, rest and repeat twice more

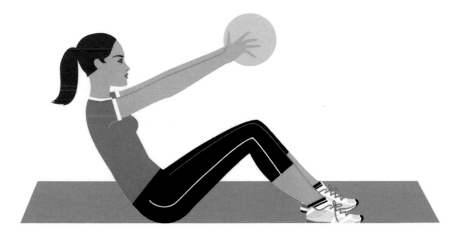

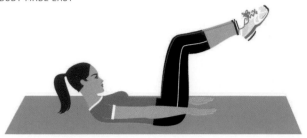

The hundred
10 reps of 10

Equipment: exercise mat
Although a basic Pilates move, this
requires effort for great results.

1 Lie on the mat with your arms
at your sides. Inhale, scooping
your belly in as you curl your head,
shoulders and upper spine off the
mat. Look down towards your
scooped belly as you exhale
deeply and draw your knees up,
one at a time, so that your thighs
form a 90º angle to the floor.
Simultaneously, lift your stretched
arms to shoulder height, parallel to
the ground, palms facing down.
2 Inhale fully into your lungs,
keeping your body stable,
supported by your abs. Beat your
straight arms vigorously up and
down 5 times, then exhale fully,
pulsing your arms another 5 times.

Roll ups
15 reps

Equipment: exercise mat
The ab roll works every part of
every abdominal muscle.

1 From the previous starting
position, squeeze your legs
and feet together as you slide your
feet away from your bottom,
keeping your soles firmly on the
mat. Inhale and scoop your belly
inwards, curling your head, neck
and shoulders off the mat until your
head and hands are reaching for
your feet.
2 Exhale fully, lengthening and
sinking your belly into your
spine to stretch your entire spine,
neck and head as you return to lie
back onto the mat.

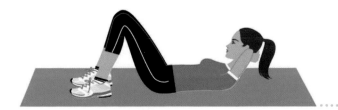

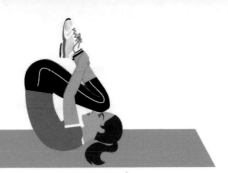

Roll with it
10 reps

Equipment: exercise mat
This massages your spine while helping to tone your thighs and stomach muscles.

1 Lie on your back. Inhale and bend your left knee, squeezing it to your chest with both hands. Curl your head, shoulders and upper body off the mat. Keep your upper body lifted, and bend forwards over your knees.

2 Exhale as you bend your right knee to your chest, holding both ankles firmly. Feet together, knees shoulder-width apart, elbows high and wide.

3 Inhale and curl your tailbone to lift your belly up and away from your hips as you roll your spine backwards, vertebra by vertebra. Use a flowing motion until you are balanced between your shoulder blades. Exhale fully as you roll back to the starting position. Keep rolling until you've finished your reps.

Cat curl
7 reps each side

Equipment: exercise mat
This will strengthen your stomach and shoulder muscles.

1 Kneel with your hands under your shoulders and knees under your hips. Inhale and arch your back up while sucking in your stomach and lowering your head.

2 Exhale and concave your back, while looking forwards.

Advanced
On the inhale, bring your right knee to your nose. On the exhale stretch your right leg out behind you.

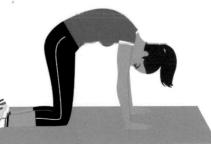

workout 3

The **lovely lower-body** workout

As with your upper body, the hourglass bottom usually just needs some toning and lifting. The following exercises will lift your buttocks by ¾in, while retaining your womanly curves.

Sexy-legs stretch
10 reps

Equipment: exercise mat
This strengthens your core, to support your back when standing.

1 Lie on the mat and pull your right knee up towards your chest, lifting your upper body as you do so. Exhale and stretch your left leg directly towards the ceiling.

2 Take hold of your left shin and extend your right leg, then switch quickly to extend your left leg. Keep you belly firmly tucked in. Breathe in, and as you exhale, switch sides once more. Repeat 5 times to complete 10 reps.

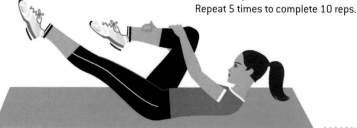

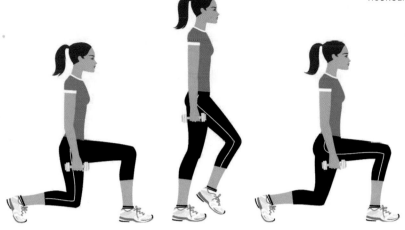

Walk of fame
22 reps

Equipment: hand weights
This walking lunge helps to define the inner thigh muscles

1 Holding weights stand with your feet hip-width apart and your knees slightly bent. Make sure your knees aren't bent over your feet. Step forward one large step and lower your back knee into a lunge position. Keep your arms loose at your sides, with your head relaxed and shoulders soft.

2 Lift your body upwards and lunge forward with the other leg. Your back leg should be bent 90°.

Dry-land swim
25 reps each side

Equipment: exercise mat
This strengthens your core, as well as elongating your arms and legs.

1 Lie on your tummy on the floor, with your legs and arms stretched out.

2 Breathe in and tighten your stomach muscles firmly. Using your stomach, bottom and thigh muscles, raise your right leg about 20cm off the floor. Hold for 1–2 seconds, then lower. Make sure your upper body isn't tensing during this move. Repeat then switch to the other leg.

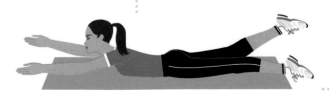

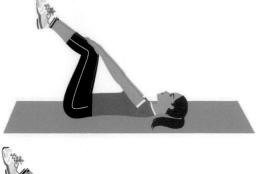

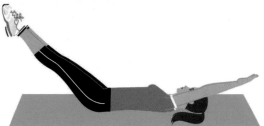

Tummy tightener
5 reps

Equipment: exercise mat
Banish that 'muffin top' and any untoned belly with this move.

1 Lie on your mat with both your knees folded into your chest. This will help stretch your thigh muscles and lower back.

2 Inhale, scooping in your belly deeply, and squeeze your legs together as you stretch them upwards. Stretch your arms up and back in a diagonal line that runs back past your ears.

3 Exhale, squeezing your lungs and belly inwards, as you circle your arms directly above your head, before pulling your knees back close to your chest.

The Iola
3 reps

Equipment: exercise mat
This stretches the tendons and tightens the belly.

1 Lie on your back and take your legs straight up, at a right angle to the floor. Flex your heels towards the ceiling, turn your feet out and take your legs out sideways into a wide V.

2 Put your hands together in a prayer position in front of your chest. Inhale and pull your abs in. As you exhale, curl your shoulders up, reaching your hands forwards through your legs. Remain in this position for 10 breaths, then return to the starting position.

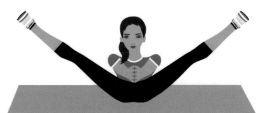

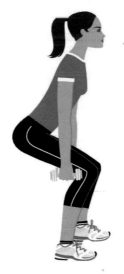

Rear rounder
15 reps

Equipment: hand weights
This easy-to-do squat will firm up
your bum, thighs and calf
muscles.

1 Stand with your feet hip-width
apart, holding the weights with
your palms facing inwards. Pull in
your tummy as you breathe in. Still
breathing in, lower your bottom
backwards and downwards, as
though you are sitting down.

2 Keep lowering yourself, but
make sure your knees aren't
over your feet. When your thighs
are parallel to the floor, pause and
exhale. Breathe in and return to the
starting position.

Let it out
15 reps each side

Equipment: exercise mat and chair
By working the quadriceps and
glutes, this move tones your
bottom and thighs.

1 Standing with your right foot
about 50cm in front of your left
foot, place your right hand on the
back of a wall. Bend your knees
until the lower part of your left leg
is parallel to the floor and the left
knee is about 5cm off the floor. Use
the chair for balance.

2 Rising back to the starting
position, kick your left leg
(with pointed toes) forwards
(no higher than your hips). Return
to starting position. Complete
your reps on this side, then repeat
on the opposite side.

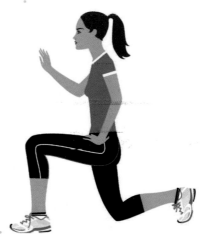

24-Hour
emergency plan

Only one day to go until you hit the beach? Still worried about fitting into your bikini? Don't worry – with this great detoxifying, tummy-flattening one-day diet you'll wow them poolside. Best of all, this diet is great for boosting your skin tone, so you'll be less likely to burn or peel.

7.00 am

Muesli (page 169) is an ideal way to start the day, as it'll keep you full for longer, so you'll be less likely to reach for a sweet treat mid morning. Plus, have a cup of organic green tea.

7.15 am

Do your workout programme, including the warm up and cool down to get your blood pumping.

8.30 am

Hit the shower and use a body brush to boost your circulation by brushing towards your heart. Add some zing to your day with a body wash that contains peppermint or eucalyptus.

9.00 am

Use a body oil straight after your shower to seal in the moisture, paying particular attention to your arms and legs, as they have fewer oil glands and so are prone to dryness.

10.00 am

Have 2 oatcakes topped with hummus to help tide you over until lunchtime, then take some time to touch up your manicure and pedicure (page 155).

11.00 am

Go for a short stroll. This will help reduce any lactic acid in your body from your earlier workout.

12.00 pm

Enjoy a warming, healthy bowl of Pomegranate Lentil Soup (page 170) for your lunch.

1.00 pm

Do some stretches (see the cool-down suggestions on page 17), then organise a massage or take a nap – but set your alarm for 2.30 p.m!

2.30 pm

Drink a refreshing glass of room-temperature water with lemon juice to help your detox along.

3.30 pm

If you're still a little peckish after your soup, fill up on a handful of omega-3-rich cashew nuts, almonds or walnuts.

5.00 pm

Get packing. If you're leaving tomorrow, don't leave all your preparation to the last minute.

6.30 pm

Try to eat your evening meal before 8.00 pm so that your body can digest it fully before you go to bed. Pile your plate high with vegetables, and add a few pine nuts or chopped almonds, or have a light meal of grilled fish with steamed vegetables.

8.00 pm

Sink into a warm bath. Add a few drops of jasmine, eucalyptus and lavender essential oils. Flick through your favourite magazine or just let your mind gently drift.

9.00 pm

If you've got an early start, make sure all your packing is done and all your documents are ready. Take a vitamin C tablet (without aspartame) with a drink of orange juice to help you absorb it, to boost your immunity if you're flying.

10.00 pm

Lights out. Sweet dreams!

Beauty **holiday** plan

Your diet's sorted, and so is your exercise programme, but what about your difficult areas? Learn about the problems you might be facing with cellulite and how to deal with them, then read how to make the most of your best bits.

Cellulite busters

Use your body brush Dry skin brushing helps to disperse cellulite deposits that have built up around the bottom and thighs. You'll have to practise brushing every day for at least one month before you see results, but it's well worth it! It really is the cheapest and easiest way to improve your bottom area.

Use some lotion Although there's no sure-fire way of eliminating cellulite with a cream, it can help to improve the appearance of your skin.

Look for products that contain caffeine and botanical ingredients such as pomegranate or grapeseed extract and aloe vera.

Drink plenty of water If you don't want to spend your hard-earned cash on cellulite treatments that may or may not deliver, reach for your kitchen tap and get drinking. About 2 litres of water each day is the quickest, easiest and most long-lasting way of beating the bumps (use a water filter if you have one).

How bad are your bumps?

There are four stages that cellulite progresses through, but whichever stage your cellulite is at right now, you can treat it to prevent it further developing into the next stage.

Stage 1 If your skin looks smooth until you squeeze it, you have 'panniculopathic' cellulite. Treat by upping your daily water intake to eliminate toxins.

Stage 2 This is 'oedemic' cellulite, where dimples are visible even without squeezing the skin. Treat by cutting out

white carbs and increasing your cardiovascular exercise.

Stage 3 When blood circulation slows down, the tissues in your skin can begin to suffer from lack of oxygen causing 'fibrotic' cellulite, which looks and feels hard and lumpy. Treat by having regular lymphatic-draining massages and a daily massage with creams that target the problem.

Stage 4 When lumps and bumps are hard and painful to touch. This is known as 'sclerotic' cellulite. See your GP.

Create those curves

If your frantic visits to the gym have not had quite the desired effects and you're still hankering for a Kylie bottom, there is hope. Just reach for the fake tan for some contouring. A tanned body instantly flatters your figure and miraculously smoothes over any bumps and lumps.

If you have trouble achieving a smooth, all-over fake-tan application yourself, Judy Naaké, self-tan guru and managing director of St Tropez, recommends salon treatment. Their bronzing-mist treatment involves two salon visits: the first session you'll be sprayed all over with St Tropez tan, and in the second visit a slightly darker colour creates contouring and shading to create long, lean limbs, a six-pack and pert bottom. 'You won't end up looking like you've overdone it, because the airbrushing mimics the same suntanning effect as the sun,' says Judy. Your contours should last around five days – long enough to inspire you to create the real thing. Best of all, the mist dries in 60 seconds so you'll look like you've had a week in Barbados before you've even packed your passport.

Before you hit the beach

1 As you have an hourglass figure, embrace your feminine shape with lots of flattering accessories: large-framed sunglasses and a floppy-brimmed sunhat; flower pins for your hair will create a stir.

2 Still haven't managed to tone those upper arms? You can do some last-minute chair dips, see Big Dipper (page 63), which will automatically tone those 'bingo wings'.

3 Remember to stand up tall. Slouching will shorten your torso and eliminate your waistline – your best feature! So, shoulders back and tummy in!

4 Sandals with a wedged heel will elongate your legs and balance out the width of your thighs. Wear them with shorts or a skirt for a happy holiday look.

5 Just 10 minutes of brisk walking will boost your metabolism and help burn off those seaside sangrias. Try walking for at least 20 minutes a day to keep your exercise programme up.

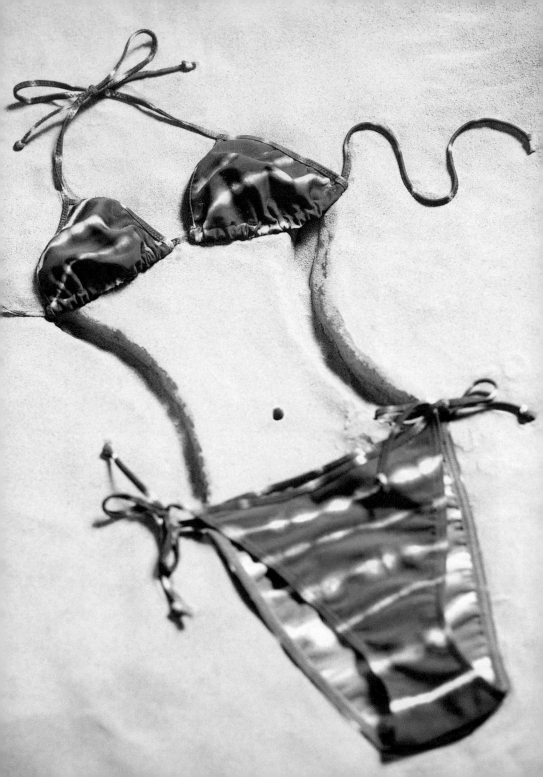

5 **Pencil** shape

You may have a straight body shape, but there's nothing boring about your figure. With the right bikini and the six-week workout plan, your body will be the best on the beach. Coupled with your healthy six-week diet plan, your energy levels and confidence will be sky high.

The **shape**

It's the figure we all probably long for: straight up and down, with no discernible hips, waist or bust. There's no denying that the pencil shape looks best in clothes – but many pencil-shaped women long for bigger busts or curvier hips. Let's face it: we girls are never satisfied with what we've got!

Your shapely characteristics

Remember, that a pencil shape doesn't necessarily mean slender: if you're carrying excess weight that settles on your bust, waist and bottom, you're also a tubular shape. It's surprising that Elle Macpherson and Dawn French are a similar basic shape: they're both straight up and down, even if their silhouettes differ slightly!

Your shoulders, waist and hips are of similar width

You have a tendency to put on weight around your waist

You have a high metabolism

Your arms, shoulders and back are shapely and toned

Your legs have little fat

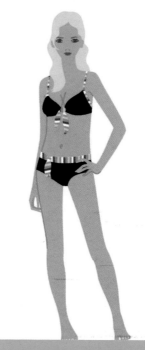

Famous pencil shapes:
Erin O'Connor
Gwyneth Paltrow

Best bikini for your shape

You've pretty much got the run of the swimwear department when it comes to choosing a swimsuit. If you are of average weight for your height, you probably don't have any part of your body to hide. So don't be afraid to go wild with creative embellishments like ruffles, jewels, ties and bows – all of which will give your straight-and-narrow physique a bit more curve and dimension. Try a padded bikini top, and when it comes to creating curves, a belted bottom is a great way to add definition to the waist and hips.

What to wear on holiday

Summer holidays are made for your shape! Short dresses and skirts, as well as boyish cutoffs are ideal. Splash out on floral prints to create a real holiday vibe and to look as different as you possibly can from your usual everyday appearance.

What to camouflage

Although you have a great figure, your lack of a waist can sometimes make you appear boxy, or wider than you really are. So pay attention to waist detail and add a belt if possible. If you wear a smock-style top, team it with heeled wedges to draw attention to your good legs.

Although there's nothing to hide per se on a pencil shape body, you can emphasise your upper body and legs to give the illusion of shape. If you're slender and pencil-shaped, choose your favourite body part to show off: if you love your legs, raise your hem; if you've got a desirable décolletage, wear tight, flattering tops that highlight your shoulders, collarbones and cleavage. Remember that when it comes to showing flesh, less is more!

Your pencil-shape diet plan

You're one of the lucky ones: you lose weight relatively easily, and evenly. So you lose weight from the top and bottom at the same time. But this doesn't mean you can rest on your (pert) behind! There is still a tendency for pencil shapes to become apple shapes if they eat too many fatty or sugary foods, so in the long term you should make sure you eat as healthily as possible and exercise regularly.

Food fact!

Personal trainer Caroline Pearce, from Power Plate UK and an ex-Gladiator, says that one of the best ways to drop weight quickly (and then to keep it off) is to check your food labels. 'Always check and monitor what you're putting into your body,' she says. 'Focus on the saturated fat and sugar content per 100g to ensure that the former is below 5% and the latter below 10% as a guide. Be aware of foods labelled "low fat" as they tend to be high in sugar to compensate. This extra, unused sugar is easily converted to fat around the stomach.'

Week-by-week
diet plan

The following diet plan is designed to help you lose any excess weight and support your workout plan. If you do not need to lose weight you can add a pudding every other day. The eating plan is to help you look and feel great, so follow it as closely as you can.

WEEK 1

Follow the 6-day Detox Plan on pages 20–21. If your BMI is in the healthy weight range, the detox week should energise you and inspire you to pump up your workouts. If your BMI is slightly over, the detox week should have achieved noticeable results – your body shape is one of the lucky ones that will lose weight fairly easily. Your list of foods to enjoy and avoid are long and short respectively: the main focus is on healthy living.

Foods to enjoy:
- Chicken • Lamb • Potatoes • Beans • Sweet potatoes
- Artichokes • Aubergines • Courgettes • Rice • Pasta
- Tomatoes • Fruit

Foods to avoid:
- White carbs (bread, pasta) • Sugar • Salt

(Avoid the above foods for health reasons, rather than weight ones. Remember that whatever your body size you should aim to eat as healthily as possible.)

WEEK 2

Our focus during the next five weeks is mostly on having a well-balanced diet that supports your workouts. This week's focus is to introduce some carbs slowly into your diet, while maintaining the focus on cleansing and detoxifying.

	BREAKFAST	LUNCH	DINNER
DAY 1	Fresh fruit salad including kiwi fruit, orange, berries, ¼ mango. Top with 65ml dairy-free yogurt, 1 tsp each of flaxseeds, pumpkin, hemp and sunflower seeds	Dairy-free Cream of Broccoli Soup (page 167)	150g tofu marinated in soy sauce. Add to ½ cup risotto rice (from a pack), with mushrooms, mangetouts and sesame seeds.
DAY 2	Porridge made with 1 cup organic porridge oats, and half soya or semi-skimmed milk/half water, plus a few prunes, and apricots	Mediterranean Roasted Vegetable Soup (page 169), with toasted rye bread or wheat-free crackers	Salad of vine tomatoes with onion, cucumber, 1 tbsp black olives, and rocket leaves
DAY 3	2-egg omelette topped with tomatoes, cheese, or red pepper	Vegetarian Flan (page 173)	50g wheat-free pasta served with 2 slices smoked salmon and 1 tsp pesto
DAY 4	2 eggs scrambled with a little milk. Add chopped chives and serve on 1 slice wholemeal toast	Three-bean Salad (page 172)	Apple, Vegetable and Quorn Curry (page 166) with wild or brown basmati rice
DAY 5	Strawberry Starter Smoothie (page 171)	Carrot and Coriander Soup (page 166)	Rice Jumble (page 171)
DAY 6	Juice 100g broccoli, 100g curly parsley, 1 apple, 2 celery sticks	Pea and Broad Bean Soup (page 170)	Ready-made wheat and gluten-free lentil and onion quiche (available from a health-food store)

WEIGHTS ARE FOR UNCOOKED PASTA AND RICE

WEEK 3

You should have noticed some weight loss by now and be feeling much more energetic. If you're a pencil shape with no weight to lose, add a wholemeal roll with your soup.

	BREAKFAST	LUNCH	DINNER
DAY 1	Juice 3 apples, 1 pear, 5mm peeled ginger	Salad of 45g brown basmati rice with ½ cup mixed vegetables. Top with 1 chicken breast, grilled	Pepper stuffed with mixture of onion, garlic and tomatoes, and 100g red lentils cooked in stock
DAY 2	Porridge made with 1 cup rolled oats and water. Add bananas, blueberries and honey (optional)	Three-bean Salad (page 172)	Clear soup made with 1 small chicken breast, Thai flavourings, pak choi, shiitake mushrooms, spring onions and tomatoes
DAY 3	1 poached egg on 1 slice of toasted wholemeal or rye bread	Salad of 1 chicken breast, griddled, raw baby spinach and rocket, plus 4 cubes feta cheese, tomato, mushrooms onion. Lemon juice dressing	Wheat-free pizza base with passata, tomato, peppers, mushrooms, pineapple, 2 slices of ham, low-fat or dairy-free cheese
DAY 4	Juice 1 celery stick, 1 carrot, 1 pear, 1 apple, 5mm peeled ginger. Blend with mixed berries, plus 1 tbsp mixed seeds	Salad of 1 rasher lean bacon, grilled and sliced, tomatoes, rocket or herb salad leaves, 50g cranberries, drizzle of balsamic vinegar	1 small chicken breast, grilled, with risotto made with basmati rice and asparagus
DAY 5	2-egg omelette with mushrooms and tomato	Salad made with 1 small can tuna, ½ avocado and sliced vegetables, salad leaves, plus 1 tbsp toasted pine nuts. Lemon juice dressing	1 chicken breast, sliced and stir-fried with mixed vegetables. Serve with brown basmati or wild rice
DAY 6	Fresh fruit salad. Add 1 tbsp crème fraîche and 1 tbsp seeds. Plus a glass of orange juice	Ready-made wheat and gluten-free lentil and red onion quiche (from a health-food store)	Small piece of monkfish fillet, grilled, with broccoli, green beans, carrots and courgette, and 1 tbsp toasted pine nuts

WEIGHTS ARE FOR UNCOOKED PASTA AND RICE

WEEK 4

You're halfway there! Keep up the good work and stick to your diet and workout plans. Don't forget to pamper yourself with a manicure or pedicure as a reward (see page 155).

	BREAKFAST	LUNCH	DINNER
DAY 1	Juice 100g broccoli, 100g curly parsley, 1 apple, 2 celery sticks. Plus 1 piece wholemeal toast with low-fat spread	1/3 block grilled marinated or smoked tofu with a salad of thinly sliced or grated vegetables	Fish in Sleeping Bags (page 167)
DAY 2	2 eggs scrambled with a little milk, on wholemeal toast, plus tomatoes and mushrooms, grilled	Vegetarian Flan (page 173)	Salad of 40g wholemeal pasta, diced cucumber, spring onions, raw mangetouts strips, cherry tomatoes and 1 small salmon fillet, grilled
DAY 3	Strawberry Starter Smoothie (page 171)	4 Ryvita, with dairy-free cream cheese, 4 slices smoked salmon, tomato and 1/2 sliced avocado	Fish in Sleeping Bags (page 167)
DAY 4	2 slices toasted rye bread with low-sugar jam, plus 1 low-fat latte and 1 glass orange juice	Carrot and Coriander Soup (page 166), with a wholemeal roll (no butter)	Marinated Chicken with Prune Salsa (page 169), with 1/2 cup brown basmati rice
DAY 5	Muesli (page 169)	Small ready-made quiche (from a health-food store)	Risotto with 1/3 block marinated or smoked tofu, grilled and cubed with green beans, onion and 4 sliced shiitake mushrooms.
DAY 6	2 Weetabix with semi-skimmed or soya milk, plus 1 banana and some strawberries	Sushi, plus miso soup (from a pack)	Stir-fried chicken with broccoli and wild rice

WEIGHTS ARE FOR UNCOOKED PASTA AND RICE

113

WEEK 5

If you feel that you've reached your goal weight, you can either stop the diet or feel free to indulge a little. If you've still got some way to go, continue with the recommended plan.

	BREAKFAST	LUNCH	DINNER
DAY 1	½ cup rolled oats made into porridge with a little milk. Serve with ½ tbsp ground flaxseeds, banana and strawberries	Soup made with stock, onion, canned tomatoes, and basil. With toasted rye bread	Roast chicken and salad of tomatoes, carrots, grated beetroot and sliced mushrooms
DAY 2	1 soft-boiled egg with 1 slice of toasted rye or wholemeal bread	Pepper stuffed with a mixture of onion, garlic and tomatoes, and 100g red lentils cooked in stock	Tuna steak, grilled, with ½ sweet potato and steamed green beans
DAY 3	Juice ⅛ watermelon, 1 kiwi fruit	Ready-made chicken and mushroom soup	Risotto made with brown basmati rice, 50g prawns, plus courgettes, peas and mushrooms
DAY 4	Blend 1 peeled and stoned mango, 1 banana, 3 tbsp low-fat yogurt, plus a handful of berries (optional)	Pitta bread stuffed with ½ avocado and 2 slices of ready-cooked chicken	1 small fish fillet (haddock or cod) grilled, with 3 small boiled potatoes and steamed green beans
DAY 5	Juice 1 celery, 1 romaine lettuce, ¼ fennel bulb, 1 orange	Salad made with 1 small can tuna, ½ avocado and a handful of rocket	Soup made with stock, onion, ½ sweet potato, leek, fresh rosemary, plus Three-bean Salad (page 172)
DAY 6	Porridge made with 1 cup rolled oats and 2 cups water. Add bananas, blueberries and honey (optional)	2-egg omelette topped with steamed spinach, sliced tomato and mushrooms	Salad of 75g wheat-free pasta shells, blanched mangetouts, halved cherry tomatoes and 1 small can tuna in spring water, drained

WEIGHTS ARE FOR UNCOOKED PASTA AND RICE

WEEK 6

Your last week! Hopefully your bad habits will be but a distant memory by now, and the healthier aspect of this diet plan will stay with you for life. Keep going — only one more week until you hit that beach!

	BREAKFAST	LUNCH	DINNER
DAY 1	Juice 1 celery stick, 100g rocket, 1 tbsp watercress, ½ avocado	Soup made with stock, ¼ squash, 1 potato, 1 onion and 2 carrots. Blend until smooth. With low-fat sour cream or 1 wheat-free roll	2 lamb chops, grilled, with 1 baked apple, mashed, red pepper, 2 boiled baby potatoes and steamed broccoli florets
DAY 2	½ cup rolled oats made into porridge with a little milk. Serve with 1 tbsp berries, 1 tsp honey and 1 tbsp seeds	1 pitta bread with 2 slices of ready-cooked turkey, ½ avocado, lettuce, tomato and 1 slice low-fat cheese	Tuna steak, grilled, with carrot and potato mash (1 potato, 3 carrots), and steamed green beans, plus salsa (spring onion, mango, celery (optional))
DAY 3	Juice 1 melon, 1 kiwi fruit, 4 pineapple chunks	Salad made with wild rice, tuna chunks and vegetables	Clear soup made with stock, 1 small chicken breast, Thai flavourings, pak choi, shiitake mushrooms, spring onions
DAY 4	2 eggs scrambled with a little milk, on 1 slice of toasted wholemeal or rye bread	Pea and Broad Bean Soup (page 170). Add harissa to taste (optional)	Salmon steak, grilled and topped with sesame seeds, mashed potatoes and steamed green beans
DAY 5	Energy Smoothie (page 167). Plus 2 pieces wholemeal toast with peanut butter	Salad of 1 boiled medium potato, lettuce, tomatoes, onion, a small can of tuna, and 1 hard-boiled egg	1 small steak, grilled and sliced, with stir-fried pak choi, shiitake mushrooms, mangetouts and spring onion. With basmati rice (optional)
DAY 6	2 eggs scrambled with a little milk, on wholemeal toast, plus tomatoes and mushrooms, grilled	1 large baked potato with 1 small can baked beans	2 small lamb chops with steamed green beans, cauliflower and courgette, plus 2 boiled baby potatoes

WEIGHTS ARE FOR UNCOOKED PASTA AND RICE

Your **six-week workout** plan

As you have a pencil body shape, and are therefore straight up and down, this workout is designed to give you some curves. Don't worry, it's impossible for you to bulk up during this six-week period, but you will find that you'll have better muscle definition and any flabby bits will be more toned.

What you'll need

Remember to check the items of equipment you will need for your workout on page 15.

Workout focus

The main focus is to strengthen and tone your body all over, while concentrating on giving you some sexy curves. If you've got some excess weight to lose (see the BMI calculation on page 12), up your cardio to help boost your metabolism with an extra 5 minutes hard burn on your body blitz.

Although your body isn't curvaceous, the pencil body shape tends to respond very quickly to workouts, so you'll be able to create contours in your arms, legs and stomach, to give you a more sculpted look.

Upper body

Your lack of bust and definition will work in your favour: you're going to concentrate on sculpting your back so that you can wear backless dresses and look fantastic in a full piece. By strengthening and adding definition to your arms, you'll look stronger as well as taller and fitter.

Mid section

With no evident waist, your body may appear stockier, or shorter, than it really is. By working on your stomach muscles, you'll trim any excess weight. The Pilates-based stomach exercises will also ensure that you're posture-perfect at all times: a move guaranteed to have you looking taller and more confident.

Lower body

Love your legs! Without a doubt, your legs are probably the envy of all your friends, so make the most of them. Concentrate on giving your legs some definition with these defining calf moves and thigh-sculpting exercises – you'll be bikini-body ready in no time!

Daily Workout Schedule

10 minutes' warm up
(See page 16.)

15-minute body blitz
Before your workout you will do a quick exercise blitz instead of interval training. Fitness consultant, Jane Wake, suggests following a varied cardio circuit for those serious about getting fit in time for their bikini-beach holiday. Since you're exercising at home, or in the park, you can choose between brisk walking, running, skipping and stair climbing. (Your step should be between 24cm and 40cm high – the higher it is, the harder you'll work.) Your suggested body blitz: 3 minutes' fairly hard cardio, 1 minute's very hard skipping, 2 minutes' very hard step-ups and 3 minutes' fairly hard jog, then repeat the whole sequence.

Weights
Each day you'll focus on a different body part: upper body, mid section, lower body. Do the recommended number of reps, but if you're finding it too easy, then increase your number of reps by 5 each week.

Day 7
This is a day of rest – a well-deserved one! If you're feeling tired and sore by Day 4, you can swap these days over, but if you time your lazy day with your 'treat' day you'll definitely feel more relaxed and pampered.

10 minutes' cool down
(See page 17.)

DAY 1
10 minutes' warm up
15-minute body blitz
Upper-body workout
10 minutes' cool down

DAY 2
10 minutes' warm up
15-minute body blitz
Mid-section workout
10 minutes' cool down

DAY 3
10 minutes' warm up
15-minute body blitz
Lower-body workout
10 minutes' cool down

DAY 4
10 minutes' warm up
15-minute body blitz
Upper-body workout
10 minutes' cool down

DAY 5
10 minutes' warm up
15-minute body blitz
Mid-section workout
10 minutes' cool down

DAY 6
10 minutes' warm up
15-minute body blitz
Lower-body workout
10 minutes' cool down

DAY 7
Rest

117

workout 1

The **shapely shoulders** workout

These moves will help you to strengthen and tone your shoulders, giving you some sexy curves. Don't worry, though, you won't bulk up, but you will appear more shapely around the shoulders and upper arms.

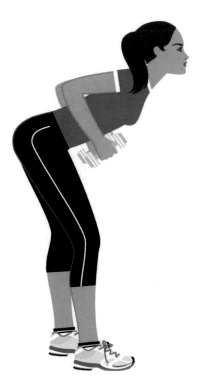

Reach out
12 reps each arm

Equipment: hand weights
Tighten up the muscles at the back of your arms with this great move.

1 Stand with your feet slightly wider than shoulder-width apart. Bend forwards from your waist, with your hips pushed back a little, so that your lower back is flat or slightly arched, torso horizontal to the floor. Keep your knees slightly flexed, and your arms hanging straight down, with a free weight in each palm.

2 Squeeze your shoulder blades together, pulling the free weights up towards your chest, elbows pointing to the ceiling, wrists in line with your forearms. Pause, then lower both arms back to the start position.

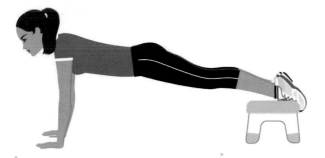

Push it
15 reps

Equipment: stair or bench
Push-ups work every muscle in
your upper body and so help to
tone arms.

1 Get down on the floor into a push-up position. Put your feet on a bench or stair, with your feet together; arms should be slightly wider than shoulder-width apart.

2 Lower yourself slowly into a full push-up position, making sure that your shoulders, hips and ankles stay in line. Lower your body as deeply as you can, pause at the bottom, then return to the start.

Having a ball
15 reps

Equipment: hand weights
and Swiss ball
This creates definition around
your shoulders and collarbone.

1 Lie face down on a bench or exercise ball with a weight in each hand. Start with your arms almost straight down, weights just above the floor.

2 Raise the free weights straight up. You should be able to feel your shoulder blades squeezing together. Pause at the top, then slowly lower the weights back to the start position, but don't let them touch the floor.

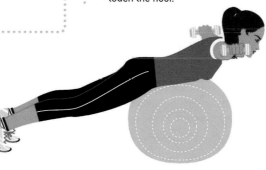

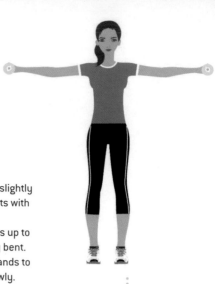

Lat raises
15 reps

Equipment: hand weights
This strengthens your upper body.

1 Stand with your feet hip-width apart, knees slightly bent. Arms by your sides, holding the weights with palms facing inwards. Stomach muscles tight.

2 Slowly raise your arms away from your sides up to shoulder level, keeping your elbows slightly bent. Palms are facing downwards; don't allow your hands to twist. Keep your torso still. Lower your arms slowly.

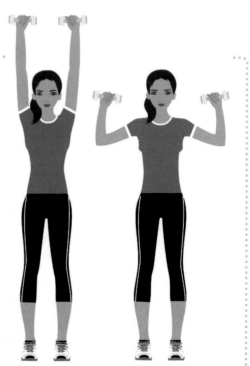

Straight up
15 reps

Equipment: hand weights
Create muscles and tone in your upper body and banish those wobbly underarm areas.

1 Stand with your feet shoulder-width apart; free weights held loosely in each hand. Raise your arms so that they are straight up in the air – on either side of your ears.

2 Pull the free weights down so that they are level to your shoulders. Hold for 1 second, then return to the start position.

The **strong-stomach** workout

Although the pencil body shape tends to have a flat stomach, it's always important to ensure that it's strong and stable so that you don't end up with lower back pain or a slightly rotund tummy. Plus, if you have any 'muffin tops', these moves will help create a waist, giving you more womanly curves.

Opposites attract
25 reps

Equipment: exercise mat
This will flatten your tummy and banish excess weight above your hips.

1 Lie on your back with your knees bent, feet flat on the floor and hands either side of your head. Lift your right foot and put onto your left knee.
2 Slowly lift your upper body, as though performing a crunch. Then turn your left shoulder and elbow up towards the outside of the opposite thigh.
Return to start and repeat the reps on that side, then work on the other.

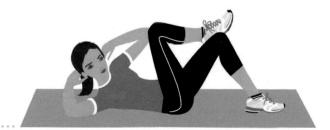

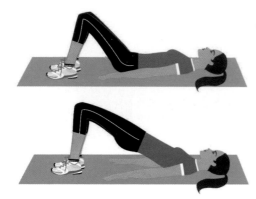

The clencher
25 reps

Equipment: exercise mat
Use your abdominal muscles to
perform this move, and keep your
hipbones lifted for optimum results.

1 Lie on your back on an exercise mat with your knees bent and your arms at your sides.

2 Breathe in, and, as you exhale, raise your pelvis towards the ceiling to around 45° to the floor. Pause, then clench your bottom muscles for the count of 2. Relax your muscles then return to the start.

Tummy tightener
25 reps

Equipment: exercise mat
Banish that little bit of
tummy just below your
belly button.

1 Lie on your mat with both your knees folded into your chest, hugging them firmly. This will help stretch your thigh muscles and lower back.

2 Inhale, scooping in your belly deeply, and squeeze your legs together as you stretch them upwards. Stretch your arms up and back in a diagonal line that runs back past your ears.

3 Exhale, squeezing your lungs and belly inwards, as you circle your arms directly above your head, then pull your knees back close to your chest.

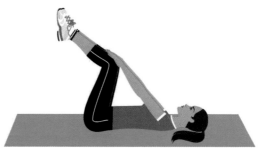

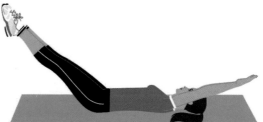

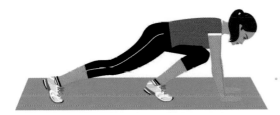

Leg and shoulders
25 reps

Equipment: exercise mat
This works those transverse muscles hard as you reach across your body.

1 Lie on your back with knees bent, hands either side of your head. Rest the calf muscle of your left leg flat against your right thigh.

2 Keep your core muscles strong; press your back against the mat. Raise your left elbow and shoulder towards your right knee. Return to the start. Do all the reps on that side then work on the other.

Tummy thrusts
30–40 reps

Equipment: exercise mat
This will your strengthen your abs, arms and legs.

1 Take a full push-up position, and focus on a spot on the mat (this will keep your neck, shoulders and head still and help you balance). Bring your right knee forward until it almost meets the right elbow. Keep your left leg extended backwards, toes pointing down.

2 Quickly return your right leg to the start position and bring your left leg forward in the same movement.

workout 3

The **lower-body** workout

Your legs are probably your best feature, so make the most of them by ensuring they're toned, cellulite-free and elongated. Squats will help you achieve the best results the fastest.

Single squat
10 reps each leg

**Equipment: exercise mat
Single squats work your thighs and bottom, giving you a toned rear.**

1 Stand with your hands on your hips, feet shoulder-width apart. Squat down on your left leg, lifting your right knee up. Squat with the left leg as low as you can.

2 Use your buttock muscles to push yourself back up. Repeat until you've completed the set, then swap legs.

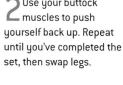

Finger on the pulse
15 reps

Equipment: hand weight (10kg – 20kg or two 5kg hand weights)A great thigh and bum toner. Make it harder by sitting back on your heels slightly when you lower your body.

1 Take one heavy hand weight and hold it with both hands. Stand with your feet slightly wider than hip-width apart, toes turned out to 45°. Squat down, making sure your heels stay flat.

2 Staying in position, pulse up and down between 8cm and 10cm for 3 seconds. Return to standing.

124

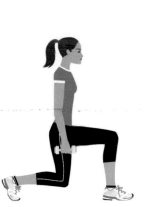
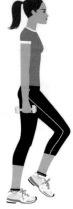
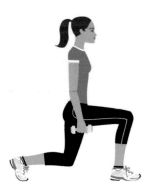

Walk of Fame
15 reps

Equipment: hand weights
There's nothing better for your legs, butt and abs than this move.

1 Holding weights, stand with your feet hip-width apart and your knees slightly bent. Make sure your knees aren't bent over your feet.

2 Step forward one step (a larger stride than you would usually take) and lower your back knee into a lunge position. Keep your arms loose at your sides, with your head relaxed and shoulders soft.

3 Lift your body upwards and lunge forward with the other leg, repeating the above movement. Your back leg should be bent 90°. Your front knee shouldn't be bent any further than your toes.

Wall flower
30 reps

Equipment: Swiss ball
A Swiss ball helps you to increase the intensity of your squat.

1 Place a Swiss ball between your lower and middle back and a wall. Keep the ball steady by pulling in your stomach muscles, with your back upright and your knees slightly forward and bent. Arms and shoulders are relaxed.

2 Slowly lower your body towards the floor until your thighs are parallel to the floor. Press your back against the ball for support. Return to the start.

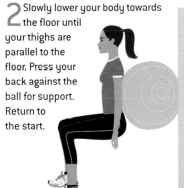

24-Hour
emergency plan

Make sure you look great when you hit the pool lounger with this detox, designed to cleanse your body and energise your mind.

7.00 am

Wake up. Our internal alarm clocks are programmed to go off after seven to eight hours sleep. So if you hit the hay at 11.00 pm last night, wake up at 7.00 am.

7.05 am

Drink a glass of lemon juice: Mix 2 tbsp freshly squeezed lemon juice (about 1 lemon), 300ml filtered water, 1 tsp maple syrup and a pinch of cayenne pepper. Transfer to a jug and add 1 cinnamon stick. Store in the fridge. This makes 4 servings so should last you through the day.

7.15 am

Skin brush then have a shower under cool water. If your skin looks tender afterwards, the temperature is too warm. Use a eucalyptus-scented shower gel for a can't-fail wake-up method, before cleansing your face with a muslin cloth.

7.30 am

Blot your hair dry; don't rub it with a towel, as this can break off damaged ends. Use a leave-in conditioner to help restore gloss. It will flatten the hair cuticles down, making your hair appear smoother.

7.45 am

Prepare yourself a bowl of porridge and honey. Use water instead of milk today.

8.00 am

Brush your teeth while standing on one leg to work your core stability muscles. This restores balance, protects your back and improves posture.

8.30 am

Time to get moving. Try yoga or a Pilates class for a gentle start. Avoid doing anything too strenuous; your body isn't ready for intense physical activity yet!

9.00 am

Drink a pint of room-temperature water. Our bodies are made up of 60% water (and our brains 70%), so it's important to keep your liquid intake up. Otherwise you may feel foggy headed or low.

10.00 am

Write out a 'to do' list. Apparently our brains are sharpest just before noon, so now's the time to get those last-minute tasks done and ticked off!

12.30 pm

Get your walking shoes on and head to the park for a fast stroll. On the way back, pick up a baked potato or a salad. Have a refreshing glass of lemon drink.

2.00 pm

Finish off your 'to do' list and reward yourself with a mint tea and a flick through your favourite magazine. Refresh yourself with a 30 minute nap.

5.15 pm

Get working! Do an entire body workout – it's the best time to achieve results.

6.00 pm

Prepare your evening meal. Try Fish in Sleeping Bags (page 167), for a filling, brain-boosting meal.

7.00 pm

Now relax. Draw a bath of warm water and add some bath salts, lavender oil and jasmine, for a mind-emptying experience. Light some candles.

7.30 pm

If you like, apply some fake tan. Make sure your skin is fully exfoliated, or try the Nutty Body Scrub (page 155). Use less fake tan on the drier areas, such as your knees and elbows.

Beauty **holiday** plan

Hurrah! Summer is finally here, so it's time to ditch those leggings in favour of some skimpy shorts. And don't worry if you're feeling a little too pale and interesting, these pointers will soon have you glowing from top to toe.

Hair do or don't

You know what havoc the sun, surf and sand can play with your locks. 'The best way to keep your hair looking sleek and healthy while on the beach is to slick it down and tie it back,' says hair guru John Frieda. Use a sun-protection hair cream or conditioning treatment and apply while the hair is wet, then secure at the base of your neck using a non-snag elastic band. Or, get creative and braid your hair. Not only will you look tantalisingly sweet and sexy but you'll also create some summery highlights in your hair.

The SPF factor

We all know that we should 'slip, slop, slap', and now researchers have found even more reason to wear sunscreen while in the great outdoors. According to the British Cancer Foundation, there are more cases of skin cancer reported each year in the UK than there are in Australia. Just 15 minutes of unprotected sun exposure can cause skin cancers, so make sure you cover up. If you're serious about protecting your skin, it makes sense to use a sun protection factor (SPF) of at least 30. Don't forget to apply cream to your ears, hands and feet – the most commonly forgotten areas. You'll still get a suntan, but

you'll achieve it without burning. Afterwards, apply a tan extender, which prolongs your tan up to nine days after being in the sun.

Fake, don't bake

A glowing tan may make you look slimmer, healthier and sexier, but, let's face it, there's nothing sexy about wrinkles! If you're lily white after winter you can still look as though you spent the colder months in tropical climes. To prepare your skin for fake tan it's important to first exfoliate dead skin cells away. This will give your skin an even, smooth surface on which to apply the cream. Then apply your fake tan cream in even strokes.

It's good to glow

Heading out on the town is a good excuse to bare some flesh. Nothing looks better than toned, tanned skin, so splurge on some flattering outfits and get ready to paint the town red! Prepare your skin by exfoliating your face and body in the shower. On your face, apply a facial exfoliant to gently wash away dead skin cells, then hold a warm washcloth to your face. This will help increase circulation and give your skin a warm, rosy glow. Wash off all the products with a blast of cold water to wake you up and add a sparkle to your skin. Spritz water all over your face and leave to dry. To replace elasticity and softness to your face, apply a deep moisturising cream to your cheeks, forehead and eye area, taking care not to pull against the skin, as this can encourage wrinkles and sagging.

Time to make up

The best part of summer is that a tan really does make you look better, so you'll need very little by way of makeup. Highlight your features, of course, but remember that less is more. Heat your eyelash curlers briefly with your hairdryer and apply to your lashes, then hold for a count of ten. Curling your lashes will give you an instant 'wide-awake' look and make your eyes look larger and more alluring.

Apply mascara to the top and lower lashes for a fantastically flirty look.

Hand check

Before you head out the door, quickly check your hands and nails. What do they look like? Are the nails nicely shaped and well maintained, or bitten to the quick? Take 10 minutes to shape and buff your nails (see page 155). Always file your nails in one direction – a sawing action will just weaken the nail and encourage breakages. Run a whitening pencil along the underside of the nail, to give the appearance of healthy, shiny nails. For a natural look, coat your nails with a ridge filler – it'll make your talons look lovely and smooth, and it contains a quick-drying agent so will take moments to apply.

Beauty must-dos

1 Is your bikini line all in check? Whisk away any unwanted hairs.

2 Avoid wearing perfume on your neck area, as this can stain your skin and cause pigmentation.

3 Don't forget to apply lip balm with an SPF to prevent blistering and dry, chapped lips.

4 Drink at least 2 litres of water every day. If you're doing a lot of physical activity, such as dancing, surfing or hiking, increase this to 3 litres.

5 Keep some dried fruits and nuts in your bag. Lack of food, mixed with long exposure to the sun can lead to sunstroke: bad for health and beauty.

6 Don't lug your makeup case out with you. All you'll need to look good from dusk till dawn is lipgloss and blotting paper.

7 Avoid fizzy drinks – alcoholic or otherwise – before the sun goes down, as you'll get dehydrated (and drunk quicker). Try a delicious, skin-friendly fruit cocktail, with mango watermelon, banana or peach instead.

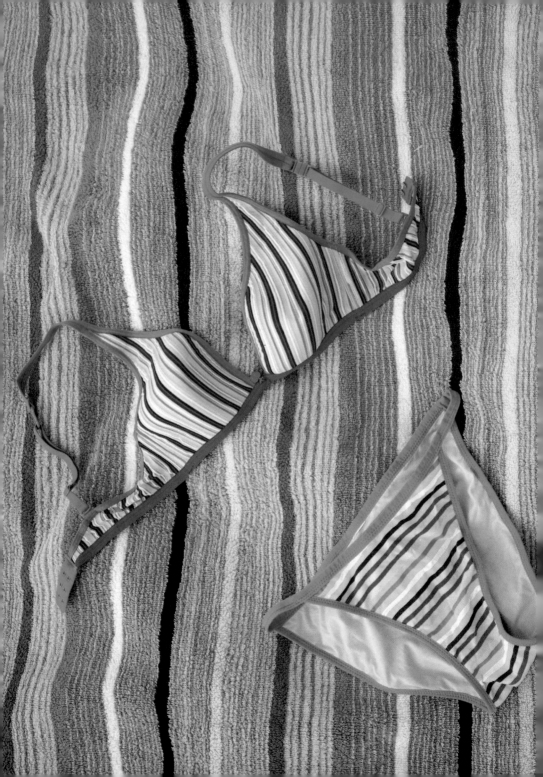

6 **Sporty** shape

Get ready to turn up the volume, because your six-week bikini diet and workout plan is all about making the most of that seriously fit body. And once you're feeling on top of the world, get yourself dressed to impress.

The **shape**

Aren't you the lucky one? There's no denying that a sporty figure is probably the healthiest and most envied shape of all. But you've worked hard for this body, so make the most of it! In just six weeks your body will look and feel the best it's ever done.

Your shapely characteristics

As you have a sporty body, you probably train or exercise regularly, and participate in several different types of sports. Your muscles are mostly well defined, and you have very few wobbly bits. A sporty body can be any of the previous body shapes (apple, pear, pencil or hourglass), but because you're so toned, it's not as easy to spot which shape you are.

You have a toned and muscular shape

You have very little body fat (less than 25 BMI – see page 12)

You are used to physical exertion

You have high energy levels

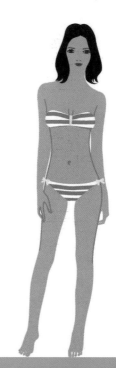

Famous sporty shapes: any Olympian, such as Dame Kelly Holmes Serena Williams

Best bikini for your shape

The world (or the swimwear section) is your oyster if you're the proud owner of a sporty silhouette. If you're intending to continue your fitness programme on holiday, then a supportive bra is a must. No matter how small your bust is, you'll still need a good sports-style bikini top.

Enhance your toned arms and shoulders with triangle bikinis, halter necks teamed with shorts-style bottoms in the brightest colours and wildest patterns you can find. If you have a small bust and would like to appear more shapely, a halter top in a bright colour will draw the eye to your chest, while the plunging front makes a focal point of your cleavage, subtly enhancing it. Triangle tops will provide the necessary lift and support that a small bust needs — look for underwired and padded tops. As for the bottoms: hipster boys' shorts-style will create curves and make your bum appear more shapely and draw attention to your hips, giving the illusion of curves.

If you want to look more feminine in your swimwear, try these touches: swimwear with frills, bows or tie sides on the bottom can add softness and subtle, flattering curves to your figure. Your shape also looks fantastic in cut-out swimsuits, where the broken-up blocks of colour and shapely, cut-out sides create gorgeous curves for a stylish poolside look.

What to wear on holiday

Make the most of your toned and taut figure, by flaunting it on the beach, by the bar and on the boardwalk. Short skirts, figure-hugging dresses and bright prints will all bring femininity to your sporty, boyish look.

What to camouflage

If you've worked hard for your taut, tight body, why hide it? However, remember that less is always more. If you're wearing a plunging neckline to show up your classic collarbone and beautiful bustline, make sure that your bottom half is slightly more demure. Team a short, flirty skirt with a less revealing top. If you're more muscular on your upper body and want to make your broad shoulders appear smaller, try loose, three-quarter-length or cap sleeves. V-neck tops or shirts with detail down the front (such as ruching or frills) will also draw the eye to the middle of your body, rather than the width on either side. For more formal occasions while abroad, try a wrap dress to emphasise your trim waist. Splash out on bold colours or prints for maximum visual impact.

Your sporty-shape diet plan

Before you begin, decide what it is you want to achieve. Do you want to build on your already great shape? Or do you want to clean up your diet a little? Or do you, despite a great body and outlook, still need to work on your confidence or beauty regime? Whichever it is, you'll find the answers in the following diet plan. Now let's get going!

Week-by-week
diet plan

After the 6-day Detox Plan you should be feeling full of energy and ready to take on the world. The following six-week diet plan is designed to help support your workout programme as well as reducing any excess bloating or water retention.

WEEK 1

Since you're probably quite healthy already, this six-week diet isn't going to be too strict. However, make sure you follow the 6-day Detox Plan on pages 20–21 before embarking on the following diet. The detox will help to ready your system for the following five-week diet and new eating plan, but the main focus is to cleanse and detox your system. This will give you extra energy and the motivation to pump up the amount of exercise you are going to do.

Foods to enjoy:
Although you should eliminate all white carbs from your diet, you're still going to enjoy lots of wholegrains, root vegetables and fruits. Red meat is off the menu to begin with, but protein such as chicken will provide your body with the energy it needs to build muscle (and lamb and pork will be introduced after the second week). And just to get you in the holiday spirit, there are loads of seafood recipes to try.

Foods to avoid:
• All white carbs (bread, pasta) • Sugar • Salt • Beef • Alcohol

WEEK 2

This week is all about maintaining the weight loss you achieved in the first week, but you're allowed a few more treats. The focus is on fresh, healthy meals that energise your body and mind.

	BREAKFAST	LUNCH	DINNER
DAY 1	Blend 100g strawberries (about 7), 100g pineapple, 1 banana. Plus 1 soft-boiled egg	85g tofu stir-fried with beansprouts, spring onions and mushrooms, served with rice noodles.	1 salmon fillet, brushed with pesto and grilled. With 50g wild rice and broccoli
DAY 2	Juice 100g celery, 50g beetroot, 100g carrots, 1 apple	Stir-fried vegetables with a handful of toasted cashew nuts, and ½ cup brown basmati rice	100g roasted chicken fillet with baked tomato, 1 large baked sweet potato and steamed runner beans
DAY 3	Juice 1 apple, 1 pear	3 crispbreads topped with 3–5 slices smoked salmon and 1 sliced tomato. Plus 1 small tub of low-fat yogurt	100g cubed pork marinated in soy sauce and lemon juice. Skewered with pepper, cherry tomatoes, mushrooms. With 1 cup of rice and a salad
DAY 4	Juice 1 celery stick, ½ avocado, 1 carrot, 1 apple	Miso soup (from a pack), plus a bowl of steamed vegetables and rice	1 chicken breast, sliced and stir-fried with green vegetables and beansprouts. If you've exercised, add ¼ cup wild or basmati rice
DAY 5	Juice 1 pear, 1 peach, 1 apple, 1 orange	Three-bean Salad (page 172)	50g basmati rice, ratatouille and a salad with feta cheese and pine nuts
DAY 6	2 eggs scrambled with a little milk, plus smoked salmon on 1 slice toasted wholemeal bread	Salad made with low-fat mozzarella, ½ avocado, tomato, salad leaves and black pepper	Soup made with stock, sliced mushrooms and mangetouts, chopped tomatoes and spring onions. Add 7 prawns. Serve with basmati or jasmine rice

WEIGHTS ARE FOR UNCOOKED PASTA AND RICE

WEEK 3

If you're finding that you're getting hungry between meals, even with your snacks, you can add a fist-sized portion of carbs. Try brown bread or rice, pulses, beans or sweet potatoes.

	BREAKFAST	LUNCH	DINNER
DAY 1	½ cup rolled oats made into porridge with half milk/half water. Plus berries and honey	Beetroot, Parsley and Feta Salad (page 166)	Salad made with 10 pieces cooked wakame, sliced, 45g brown basmati rice, soya beans, cucumber, carrot, mangetouts, sesame seeds
DAY 2	Juice ½ grapefruit and ½ cucumber, then add the juice of 1 lemon. Serve on ice with chopped mint (optional)	Salad of ½ grapefruit (in segments), with a handful of rocket and the seeds and juice of 1 pomegranate	1 fish fillet (haddock or cod), grilled, plus salsa made with lemon juice, tomato, 2 chopped anchovy fillets, 8 chopped black olives, garlic, parsley. With sweet potato mash and green beans
DAY 3	Juice 100g each peeled and chopped celeriac, celery, peeled Jerusalem artichoke. Plus mint	A sauce of onion, ½ can tomatoes and sliced mushrooms. With 70g wheat-free pasta and basil	Soup made with stock, leek and mushrooms, topped with 50g chopped ready-cooked chicken
DAY 4	1 boiled egg with 1 slice toasted wholemeal bread. Plus 1 glass orange juice	Miso soup (from a pack), plus 4 Ryvita topped with dairy-free cream cheese, smoked salmon pieces, sliced tomato	Lamb with Aubergine and Raisins (page 168), with couscous
DAY 5	Juice 3 peaches, 2.5cm peeled root ginger, 1 apple	2 slices of lettuce, cherry tomatoes, ½ sliced avocado and 2 thin slices of cheese on crispbreads or rye bread	½ can tuna chunks with 1 cup steamed mixed vegetables, and ½ cup brown basmati rice
DAY 6	Juice 1 lettuce and ½ peeled lemon, then stir into 100ml chamomile tea	Pea and Broad Bean Soup (page 170)	Thai Green Curry with Prawns (page 172), with brown basmati rice

WEIGHTS ARE FOR UNCOOKED PASTA AND RICE

WEEK 4

Take your measurements this week. You may not notice much difference in inch loss, but you should find that you feel less bloated and your upper arms and thighs may be slimmer.

	BREAKFAST	LUNCH	DINNER
DAY 1	1 poached egg on 1 slice of toasted wholemeal bread. Plus 1 glass orange juice	3–4 slices ready-cooked chicken with a salad of herb or rocket leaves, 100g sprouting beans, spring onions, ½ sliced avocado	1 tuna steak, grilled, with broccoli, green beans and 2 boiled baby potatoes
DAY 2	Energy Smoothie (page 167). Plus 1 piece wholemeal toast with jam or peanut butter	40g sliced ready-cooked lamb with salad of baby spinach (steamed or raw), ½ cup brown basmati rice, 2 dates, 1 tbsp sultanas	Minestrone Soup (page 169) with 1 wholemeal roll. Plus fresh fruit salad with 1 tbsp crème fraîche
DAY 3	Fresh fruit salad with a small tub of low-fat yogurt and 1 tbsp mixed ground seeds	½ can tuna with a salad of ½ sliced avocado and ½ cup wholemeal couscous	Miso soup (from a pack). Plus pepper stuffed with mixture of onion, garlic and tomatoes, and 100g red lentils cooked in stock
DAY 4	Juice ½ melon, 1 apple, 1 celery stick	Soya Bean Salad (page 171)	Tuna steak, grilled, with steamed purple sprouting broccoli and vegetables, plus brown basmati rice
DAY 5	Juice 100g cauliflower, 2 apples, 200g carrots, 1 large tomato	Wild rice with salmon chunks and a salad of peppers, ½ avocado, spring onions and tomatoes	Mediterranean Roasted Vegetable Soup (page 169)
DAY 6	½ cup rolled oats made into porridge with half milk/half water, with a little honey, berries and 1 tbsp mixed sunflower and pumpkin seeds	Tortilla wrap with 3 thin slices of ready-cooked chicken, ½ avocado and lettuce. Add lemon juice and pepper	Fish in Sleeping Bags (see page 167)

WEIGHTS ARE FOR UNCOOKED PASTA AND RICE

WEEK 5

Well done, you've finished four weeks of a strict bikini diet. If you feel that you've lost enough weight, you can finish the diet here. Otherwise, carry on for the next two weeks.

	BREAKFAST	LUNCH	DINNER
DAY 1	Juice ½ grapefruit, ½ fennel bulb, 100g celery	½ cup wholemeal couscous, cooked and tossed with a raw salad of celery, sultanas, spring onions, peppers, mushrooms and tomatoes	Lime, Tomato and Scallop Salad (see page 168)
DAY 2	Juice 125g papaya, 125g cucumber, 2 oranges,	2-egg omelette with 1 sliced tomato and 4 mushrooms. Plus 1 small pot of low-fat yogurt	1 small salmon fillet, grilled, with ½ cup brown basmati rice and 1 cup steamed mixed vegetables
DAY 3	1 cup rolled oats made into porridge with a little milk, plus 1 tsp honey, ½ cup berries and 1 tbsp mixed seeds	Pitta bread filled with 3–4 slices ready-cooked chicken, lettuce leaves and ¼ sliced or mashed avocado. Plus 1 small tub of low-fat yogurt	Carrot and Coriander Soup (page 166) Spaghetti Bolognese (made according to pasta-pack recipe) with wheat-free pasta
DAY 4	Juice 1 orange, 1 pear, 1 apple, 5mm peeled ginger	Three-bean Salad (page 172)	Stir-fry 250g mixed vegetables with 40g prawns. Serve with noodles
DAY 5	2 eggs scrambled with a little milk, plus 2 slices of smoked salmon on 1 slice of toasted wholemeal or rye bread	Minestrone Soup (page 169)	50g lamb, cubed. Skewered with quarters of eating apple, mushrooms, cherry tomatoes, peppers, onions and grilled
DAY 6	Juice 1 kiwi fruit, 1 apple, 1 pear, 5mm peeled ginger	50g tofu, marinated in soy sauce and grilled, with 1 cup steamed mixed vegetables and ½ cup brown basmati rice	Soup made with stock, ¼ cubed squash, 1 chopped potato, onion and 2 carrots. Cook until soft, then blend. Serve with 1 slice of toasted rye bread

WEIGHTS ARE FOR UNCOOKED PASTA AND RICE

WEEK 6

Hurrah! You're almost there! This week is about continuing all your hard work, with lots of protein and cleansing drinks to make sure you look the best you possibly can on that beach.

	BREAKFAST	LUNCH	DINNER
DAY 1	1 poached egg with 1 slice of toasted wholemeal bread	Salad made with lettuce, baby spinach and rocket, mixed chopped or grated vegetables, tomatoes, spring onions. Add 75g feta cheese and a lemon juice dressing	1 tuna steak, grilled, with ½ cup green beans, a handful of baby spinach and ½ cup brown basmati rice
DAY 2	Juice 1 grapefruit, 1 apple, 1 celery, 1 pear, 1 kiwi fruit	Sliced onion cooked in ½ tbsp oil with 4 cherry tomatoes and sliced mushrooms. Add ½ can tuna, flaked. Heat through. Toss with 40g wheat-free pasta	Soup made with stock, leek, 1 potato and 10 sliced mushrooms, with toasted rye bread
DAY 3	Fresh fruit salad with 1 tbsp mixed sunflower, pumpkin and flax seeds	Stir-fry 1 cup of mixed vegetables with 1 tsp sesame seeds. Toss with 25g glass noodles	½ small turkey breast, steamed, with sweet potato mash (1 sweet potato, 2 carrots) and green beans
DAY 4	½ cup rolled oats made into porridge with half milk/half water, with 1 tsp honey, ¼ cup berries, 1 tsp flaxseeds	1 sushi selection and a bowl of miso soup (from a pack)	55g wheat-free pasta with a sauce made with onion, fried in a little oil, ½ can chopped tomatoes, ½ tbsp pesto and ½ garlic clove
DAY 5	Juice of 3 oranges blended with 3 handfuls mixed berries	Steam 1 cup mixed vegetables and mix with soy sauce, ½ cup brown basmati rice, 1 tsp sesame seeds	Clear soup made with 1 small chicken breast, Thai flavourings, pak choi, shiitake mushrooms, spring onions
DAY 6	½ can baked beans on 1 slice toasted wholemeal bread, plus a little grated cheese	Carrot and Coriander Soup (page 166)	1 chicken breast, stir-fried with soy sauce and 1 tsp honey, 1 tbsp sesame seeds. With mixed vegetables

WEIGHTS ARE FOR UNCOOKED PASTA AND RICE

Your **six-week workout** plan

As you're already a fitness enthusiast, this programme is about working your body even harder, to make it leaner and more toned, and to further increase your fitness levels. If you find that the workouts don't challenge you enough, add an extra 5 reps to each move every week, and feel the burn!

What you'll need

Remember to check the items of equipment you will need for your workout on page 15.

Workout focus

Although you're already super-fit and toned, you don't want to add any more bulk to your body – just increase your level of fitness and push yourself a little harder. 'If you become complacent in your workout, then your body shape won't improve,' says personal trainer BJ Rule. 'Try different types of workouts to vary your exercise, and to keep your mind active and interested.'

Upper body

These exercises will concentrate on toning and tightening your arms and upper body, so that you can wear the brightest bikini on the beach. Watch out Baywatch, here you come! You'll also do some upper-back strengthening and toning work, to help balance out your sporty lower half.

Mid section

There is a killer-abs workout for you in this section. It's hard, but the results will be well worth it. Make sure you follow the instructions carefully, as sporty figures can suffer from related injuries, such as lower-back problems or pulled muscles.

Lower body

Your perky bottom is probably your favourite body part, so make sure it's bikini-ready with this workout. Add some leg-lengthening exercises (sporty types can sometimes appear squat or shorter than they really are) and you're ready to hit that beach.

Daily Workout Schedule

10 minutes' warm up
(See page 16.)

20–30 minutes' interval training
You're no stranger to the gym, so your workout is all about increasing your body strength and endurability. If you can jog for 20 minutes before exhausting yourself, then start off with 20 minutes of interval jogging on the first day (1 minute jog, 1 minute very fast sprint). If you're very fit, boost this first day's exercise to 30 minutes of the same type of interval training. You will also be doing swimming and cycling during your week's interval training – follow the timings on the chart (right).

Weights
Each day you'll focus on a different body part: upper body, mid section, lower body. Do the recommended number of reps, but if you're finding it too easy, then increase your number of reps by 5 each week.

Day 7
This is a day of rest – a well-deserved one! If you're feeling tired and sore by Day 4, you can swap these days over, but if you time your lazy day with your 'treat' day you'll definitely feel more relaxed and pampered.

10 minutes' cool down
(See page 17.)

DAY 1
10 minute's warm up
20 minutes' run
Upper-body workout
10 minutes' cool down

DAY 2
10 minutes' warm up
15 minutes' fast swim
Mid-section workout
10 minutes' cool down

DAY 3
10 minutes' warm up
20 minutes' cycle
Lower-body workout
10 minutes' cool down

DAY 4
10 minutes' warm up
30 minutes' swim
Upper-body workout
10 minutes' cool down

DAY 5
10 minutes' warm up
30 minutes' run
Mid-section workout
10 minutes' cool down

DAY 6
10 minutes' warm up
30 minutes' cycle
Lower-body workout
10 minutes' cool down

DAY 7
Rest

workout 1

The **sporty-spice upper-body** workout

You're already the proud owner of a strong upper body. These moves will just help you to continue your toning programme.

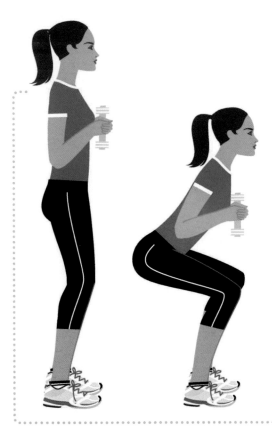

Sporty squat
30 reps

Equipment: hand weight (at least 10 kgs)
This is a great exercise for your upper arms and shoulders, plus it has the added bonus of toning up your thighs.

1 Hold the weight to your chest and lower your body into a squat.

2 Hold, then, using your thighs, lift yourself back into a standing position. Repeat three sets of 10.

Sporty swing
30 reps

Equipment: hand weight (at least 10 kgs)
This works on the previous move, but
engages your stomach muscles more.
It may look easy, but you'll definitely feel
it tomorrow!

1 Standing with your feet apart, hold the weight between your legs.

2 Swing it back and forth until you have momentum going. Swing the weight backwards and forwards, flicking the weight out towards the front when it's at its highest point in front of you.

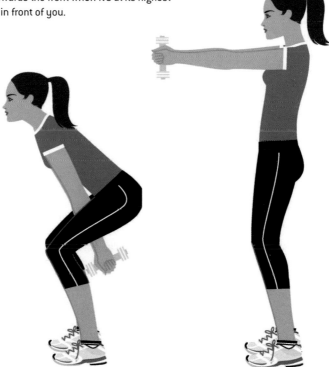

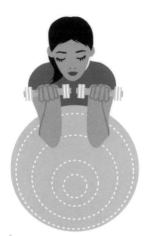

Sporty lift
30 reps

**Equipment: hand weights
(at least 5 kgs)**
**A great all-over upper body workout. This works
your arms, shoulders and upper back.**

1 Holding the weight, lift it above your head, making sure that your arm is vertical from your shoulder and behind your ears. Don't lock your arm and make sure you don't sway.

2 Return to the start position and repeat then repeat with the other arm.

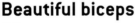

Beautiful biceps
30 reps

Equipment: Swiss ball and hand weights
Work on those biceps for alluring, toned upper arms. Pull your stomach muscles in tight to avoid straining your lower back.

1 Lie on an exercise ball, so that you're kneeling in front of it, with your feet shoulder-width apart. Keep your back straight and your belly button tucked tightly in. Hold a weight in each hand and rest your arms at your sides. Extend your arms straight ahead of you, palms facing upwards.

2 Bend your elbows and lift the weights towards your shoulders, then lower them again. Return to the starting position.

3 Turn your palms towards each other, slightly bend your elbows and raise your arms outwards, so that your hands are at shoulder height. Lower back to starting position.

workout 2

The **sporty stomach** workout

If you've already got a six-pack, these moves will be easy for you, so double the number of reps for a more challenging workout.

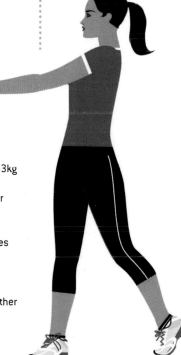

Boxing Day

5 reps
(increasing with
practise and strength)

Equipment: medicine ball
Keeping your stomach muscles taut
and strong, this move goes a long way
to helping build and enhance that six-pack.

1 Stand side on to a wall, 1–2m away, and holding a 2–3kg
medicine ball. Rotate towards the wall, engaging your
core muscles and throwing the ball against the wall. Power
your throw from your stomach muscles, not your arms.
2 Catch the ball without having to run after it — the
movement needs to be sure and controlled. Swap sides
after a few throws.

Advanced

The fitter and more practised you get at this move, the further
away from the wall you can move.

Boat race
30 seconds hold

Equipment: exercise mat
Using strength and balance, you'll be engaging your stomach muscles to banish any little pot belly.

1 Sit on your sitting bones and grab the underside of your knees. Walk your toes in to your buttocks. Draw your shoulder blades down into your back, lifting your chest at the same time.

2 Holding your legs, keep your back straight and pull your stomach muscles in. Straighten your legs up until your toes are level with your eyes. If you can, release your arms and hold them in front of you. Hold this position for 30 seconds, then return to the start.

Stomach strengthener
30 seconds hold

Equipment: exercise mat and Swiss ball
This is a lovely stretch for your upper body and back, while you're working on strengthening those stomach muscles.

1 With your knees on the floor, rest your elbows on a Swiss ball. Extend your legs to a plank position, supporting your weight with your arms and keeping your body flat and spine neutral by engaging your core abdominals.

2 Try to hold for 30 seconds, but stop if you feel tired.

Advanced
Increase the intensity by breathing in, then as you exhale, roll the ball forward, keeping your feet still. Inhale and roll the ball back to the start.

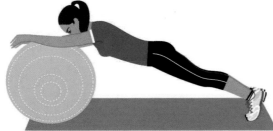

The clencher

5 reps

Equipment: exercise mat
Tone your buttocks as well as your midriff with this basic Pilates move. It might look basic, but it really works your tummy.

1 Lie on your back on an exercise mat with your knees bent and your arms at your sides.

2 Breathe in, and, as you exhale, raise your pelvis towards the ceiling to around 45° to the floor. Pause, then clench your bottom muscles for the count of 2. Relax your muscles then return to the start position.

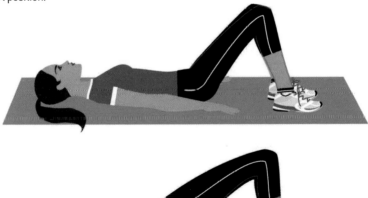

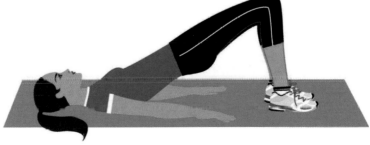

Pump it up
15 reps

**Equipment: exercise mat
A great workout for your
abdominal and transverse
muscles (that run either side of
your belly button). Take it slowly
for best results.**

1 Lie flat on the floor and lift your
legs 90º to your body.

2 Keep your core muscles
engaged and gradually bend
your legs, keeping your thighs
where they are, but moving your
feet in an arc until they touch your
bottom. Return your legs to the start.

Advanced
If you find the above move easy, try
this tummy tightener. Extend your
legs fully until they are hovering
about 3–5cm off the floor, then bend
and return to the vertical position.
Make sure you're not lifting your
lower back off the floor – all the
effort comes from your stomach
muscles.

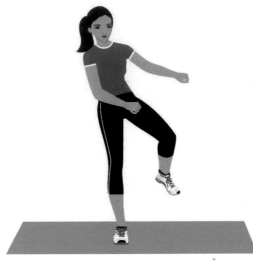

Speed skater
30–60 seconds

**Equipment: exercise mat
These moves offer a great core
workout by forcing you to use
your core muscles to control
your balance.**

1 In a standing position, feet
hip-width apart, hop to the right
into a one-legged squat, bending
your left knee and swinging your
arms to the left, like a speed skater.
Hop to the left, bending your
right knee and swinging your arms
to the right.

2 Make sure your stomach
muscles are tightened and your
pelvic floor muscles are pulled
upwards. Repeat this exercise for at
least 30 seconds, working your
way up to 1 minute as you perfect
your move.

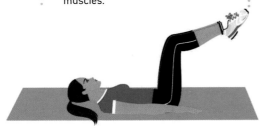

workout 3

The **fit and firm** workout

These moves will ensure that your legs remain long, thin and shapely and don't bulk up. Avoid using leg weights – instead, squats and leg lifts are best.

Kangaroo
2 minutes each leg

Equipment: bench or bed
Your hamstrings and glutes will thank you for this move.
It's a hard one, but gives you quick results.

1 Kneel on all fours on the surface of your bed or bench. Keep your knees on the edge and face towards the centre, with your hands directly below your shoulders and your knees below your hips. Keep your spine straight and neutral.

2 Straighten your right leg behind you and lower it towards the floor, so that your toe is just touching the floor. Keeping your right leg straight and heel flexed, toes pointing towards the floor, lift it directly up towards the ceiling for a count of 2 until it's level with your hips. Lower to the starting position for the count of 2. Repeat for 2 minutes with your right leg, then repeat for the other leg.

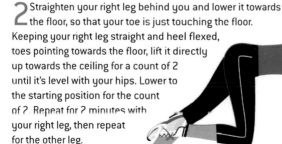

Box squat
30 reps

Equipment: hand weights
Create some definition and banish any excess
weight on your back with this beautiful back
toner.

1 Stand with your feet hip-width apart and a weight in each hand by your sides. Slowly squat down as though you're going to sit on a chair.

2 As you squat, raise the weights straight up in front of you to shoulder height, keeping your arms straight and your palms facing the floor. Return to the start and repeat.

Advanced
Try lifting one foot until your toes are flexed on the floor, and hold while you squat and lift your arms. Repeat on the other leg.

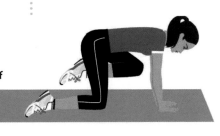

Kangaroo hop
30 reps each leg

Equipment: exercise mat
Tighten those inner thighs and give yourself
a bottom lift at the same time.

1 Kneel on the floor on all fours, with your stomach muscles pulled tight, and your back flat. Pull your right knee into your chest, then push it back out behind you in a slow, controlled movement, until it's completely straight and parallel to the ground.

2 Return to the start and complete your reps on this side, then repeat on the opposite side.

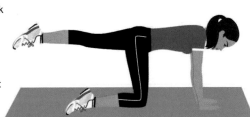

Scrambled eggs
25 reps

Equipment: exercise mat
Tighten those inner thighs and elongate your legs with this brilliant move. Keep your body still and don't let your tummy muscles sag.

1 Kneeling on all fours, straighten out your left leg behind you, level with your hips and with your heel flexed, so that it's parallel to the wall.

2 Keeping your leg high (but no higher than your bottom), swing it out sideways in a slow, controlled movement. Make sure you don't overbalance or tilt your back. Return to the start and complete your reps on this side, then repeat on the opposite side.

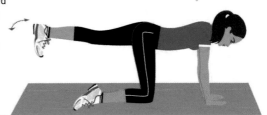

Helicopter
30 seconds each leg

Equipment: exercise mat
Make sure you keep your upper body firm and still and you'll see the results in your bottom very quickly.

1 From the same starting position as above, move your left leg out to the side, level with your hip, making sure your heel remains flexed.

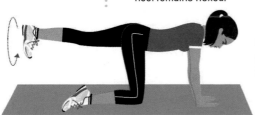

2 Rotate your leg in very small circles: 30 seconds in each direction. Return to the start position and repeat your reps on the opposite side.

24-Hour
emergency plan

Leaving for your holiday tomorrow and still have jiggly bits?
Tighten those thighs and 'muffin tops' with this emergency plan.

7.00 am

Start your morning with a warm glass of water with lemon juice. Whiz up a healthy berry juice: squeeze the juice from 3 oranges and blend with a handful each of strawberries, blueberries and raspberries.

7.30 am

Before you get in the shower use a loofah all over your body. Begin at your toes and brush your skin upwards towards your heart. This will help boost your circulation and improve the appearance of your skin.

8.00 am

Deep-cleanse your hair with a pH-balancing shampoo. Apply a leave-in conditioner. Before drying off, use an ultra-moisturising body oil all over, paying particular attention to the soles of your feet and your elbows.

9.00 am

Don your fitness gear and get moving. Begin with a 15 minute warm up then follow the workout for your body shape. Remember to cool down with your 10 minute stretches. Follow with your morning snack. Add 1 tsp of miso to boiling water.

11.00 am

Make sure your eyebrows, bikini line and any other errant hairs are waxed, plucked or bleached. Now apply a deep moisturising face mask and lie down while it does its work for 30 minutes. Rinse and apply your usual toner, moisturiser and eye cream.

3.30 pm

Avoid any last-minute stress by sorting out your holiday wardrobe.

12.00 pm

Choose one of the lunches from the 6-day Detox Plan on pages 20–21.

1.00 pm

It's time for another workout – pop in a yoga or Pilates DVD for some gentle stretching.

4.30 pm

Hit the shops! Not only will you avoid last-minute splurging at the airport but you'll also make sure you have everything you need to look fabulous and fit every day of your holiday.

2.00 pm

An afternoon sleep has been shown to improve your circulation, boost your brainpower and even make you thinner. So head to your bedroom, put on your eye mask and allow your thoughts to drift, but don't forget to set your alarm clock for 3.00 pm.

6.00 pm

Enjoy a light, nutritious dinner of steamed vegetables, rice and your choice of fish. Try salmon for its abundance of omega-3 fatty acids, which are great for smooth, glowing skin.

9.00 pm

Give yourself a foot and hand massage with a lavender-infused moisturiser. This will help you sleep well, and give you silky-soft mitts and tootsies.

3.00 pm

Wakey wakey! Remove your eye mask. Put on some holiday music, to get you in the mood. Re-energise yourself by drinking a sparkling water with grated fresh root ginger and a squeeze of lemon – this will help support your liver and kidneys, as they continue to detox.

10.00 pm

Time for bed. Do some stretching (see page 17) to relax your muscles, then hop into bed and turn off the light.

Beauty **holiday** plan

Now that your body is fit, buff and beautiful, it's time to get it bikini-ready on the outside with some pampering.

Max the moisture

As a sporty type, you're probably in and out of the swimming pool, or showering at your gym. Although all that exercise is fantastic for your body, it may leave your hair dry and split, and your skin crying out for some moisture. Try these top-to-toe beauty treatments:

Hair treatment

Invest in a good-quality hair restorative treatment. If you're unsure which one is best for you, speak to your hairdresser. Many products now contain a sun protection factor (SPF), so you can protect your hair while outdoors. This is particularly important when you're on holiday and out in the sun more often than usual.

How to apply hair treatments

Wash your hair with a deep-cleansing shampoo, then apply the deep-conditioning treatment from the roots to the tips, using a wide-toothed comb to untangle any knots and spread the mixture evenly. For extra-deep conditioning, pop a shower cap on your head, as this will keep in the heat and activate the conditioner. (Or you can use a heated towel.) Either lie back in your bath and allow the warm water to soothe your muscles, or, if you're showering, spend the time giving yourself a manicure and pedicure (right).

Moisture mask

Outdoor sports may be great for your body, but your skin may be paying the price. Lucy Russell, founder of Lucy Russell Organics (www.lucyrussellorganics.co.uk) recommends applying a yogurt mask to brighten tight, dry skin. 'The natural lactic acid in the yogurt helps to dissolve dead skin cells and draw out impurities from the skin,' she says. Lucy also recommends that you apply a thin layer of organic full-fat natural yogurt to your face and neck (avoiding the delicate eye area). Leave for about 5 minutes, or until the mask has dried. Remove the mask with your normal cleanser and a cotton flannel or muslin cloth soaked in hand-hot water.

Beauty fact!

Mama Mio's Tanya Kazeminy Mackay says that massaging thighs and tummy with cream for at least 20 seconds each day can help to break up fatty deposits.

Body prep

Your body may be fit and toned, but is it smooth and soft? Beautician Joyce Connor, owner and founder of Brides and Beauty (www.bridesandbeauty.co.uk) recommends you give yourself a full-body exfoliation to remove all dry skin and to give your skin a polished look. 'A weekly scrub in the shower is very invigorating, as it boosts your circulation and is necessary before applying fake tan,' she says. Use a specially formulated body scrub, or try Joyce's homemade recipe:

Nutty body scrub

Whiz 100g ground nuts (try almonds or flaxseeds), 50g oatmeal and 50g wholewheat flour in a blender until reduced to a coarse mixture. Pour into a glass jar with a screw top. To use, scoop out a handful and put it into a bowl, then add enough water to make a paste. Rub over your body to loosen any dry or flaking skin. Store the mixture in the fridge and use within 1 month, or it can be frozen and used within 3 months.

The perfect pedicure and manicure

1 Trim your toenails neatly, straight across the top, without going too short.
This is a more attractive shape and helps prevent ingrowing toenails. Continue with the same routine as the manicure.

2 Wash your hands and gently scrub your nails, then dry your hands thoroughly.

3 File and shape your nails using a gentle stroke. Avoid the corners of your nails, as this can weaken them. If you're going to be doing lots of ball activities, or spending a lot of time in the water, it's best to keep your fingernails fairly short.

4 Apply a softener to all your cuticles and place your hands in warm water for a few minutes, then gently push back the cuticles revealing the half moons.

5 Apply hand lotion and massage the palm of one hand with the thumb of the other. Work your way over the remainder of the hand.

6 Wrap an orange stick with cotton wool. Dip into nail-polish remover and rub over the nail to remove any residue.

7 Choose a bright, summery colour for your holiday nails. Paint one stroke down the centre of your nail then stroke the sides until the nail is covered.

8 Allow to set for a minute or so before applying the second coat of polish.

9 Wait until the polish is dry to the touch and then apply the top coat.

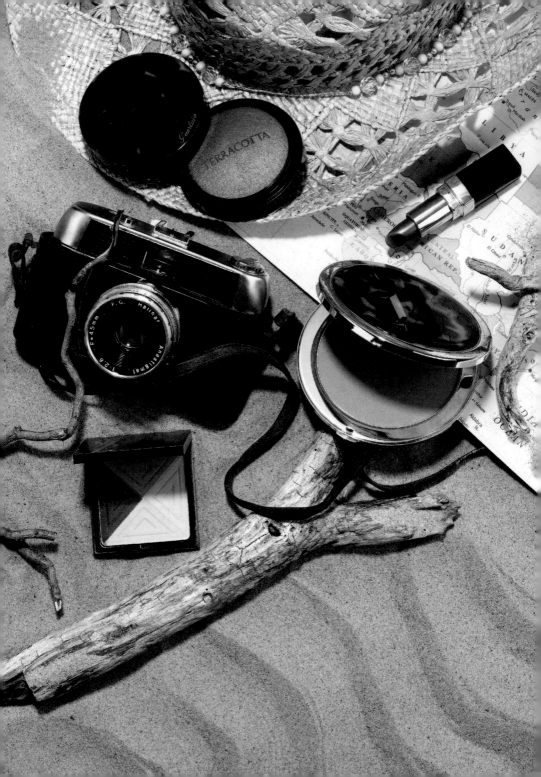

7 **On** holiday

Hurrah! You're finally there! Whether you're on a sandy beach in the Bahamas, or trying to get comfortable on the pebbles in Brighton you should be feeling very proud of yourself. Six weeks of hard work, and you look fabulous! It's your holiday, so kick back, relax and enjoy your well-earned rest.

Your **holiday diet**

Don't let all your hard work go down the drain. You can still enjoy the sun, sand and sangrias while keeping healthy. Even a few changes can make the difference between returning home feeling revitalised or returning home with excess bodily baggage.

For breakfast

Enjoy some protein in the morning, such as a poached or boiled egg, followed by a small tub of low-fat yogurt or a small bowl of fruit salad. Avoid the fruit juices, as you can't be 100% sure that they're freshly squeezed (they're usually from a carton and full of sugar) and drink warm water with lemon juice instead. You can still enjoy tea and coffee – it'll add to your daily water intake.

Foods to enjoy

Fresh fruit The best thing about buffets is you can load up on the good stuff. So go mad on the fruit counter and reach for the darkest coloured fruit. The darker it is, the more nutrients it will contain.

Yogurt Most buffets will provide a low-fat version of yogurt, but if they don't, just eat sparingly.

Water Keep your glass topped up to replenish liquid lost through heat, air-conditioning and alcohol.

Foods to avoid

Bacon It's usually fried and sits soaked in fat.

Sausages Laden with fat, sausages have very little nutritional value.

Cheese and ham All cheese and ham is high in fat and salt, and processed versions are particularly worth avoiding. But if you want to enjoy a little of the regional cheese or ham occasionally, practise your school-level languages and ask the locals for their deli recommendations.

Bread and pastries Avoid the bread basket, unless there's wholemeal bread or rolls on offer. Although croissants are tempting, let's face it, they contain very little goodness and a lot of fat. Save these for a one-off treat.

For lunch

Most lunches while you're on holiday tend to be sandwiches, burgers or chips – all fat- and carb-laden meals. Take advantage of your location and enjoy some of the local delicacies. For example, a Greek salad without the dressing is low in fat and full of flavour, containing salad leaves, tomatoes, olives, feta cheese and spring onions. Just ask for it sans dressing and add a little of your own olive oil and the juice from a wedge of lemon. Of course, if you're hankering after those fries that look and smell delicious, then order some. Just keep to a small portion (a starter size is usually enough) and avoid adding extra salt. It is your holiday after all – just keep your indulgences in moderation.

Soups Many European countries make delicious chilled soups (such as gazpacho), which are full of nutrients.

Antipasto, mezze and pasta When it comes to antipasto or mezze, choose just a small selection as a tasty starter (you can always blot it with a napkin if it is very oily), and eat it only every other day, or choose a few olives instead. Eat as the Italians do and enjoy just a small plate of pasta. Avoid adding extra oil or salt.

Foods to avoid

Bar food tends to be grilled, fried or laden with fat. If you really can't find a healthy alternative, then order a burger and remove the bun before eating.

Chips The same applies here, but thick potato wedges are less calorific than skinny fries, and you might also find sweet potato wedges, which are a healthier alternative.

Crisps Laden with salt, crisps will add pounds as well as causing you to retain water, making you look bloated.

Bar snacks Although a handful of nuts is good for you, salty peanuts are a different matter entirely – avoid, and enjoy some olives instead.

Foods to enjoy

Salads It's your holiday, you're on the beach and it's a scorcher, the last thing you want is hot, fried food, so enjoy as many salads as possible. If you're in a country where it's essential to avoid tap water, avoid salads and eat plenty of veggies, but make sure they're cooked first.

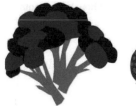  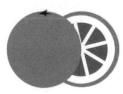

For dinner

If you're on a beach holiday, seafood will undoubtedly make up a large proportion of your dining menu. Eating fish as much as possible for your evening meal is the easiest way to keep to your healthy eating plan, while still enjoying a night out.

Foods to enjoy

Fish, fish and more fish Tuna, mackerel, swordfish: the sea is your oyster, so dive into the wonderful selection you will find! Ask for your fish to be grilled and served with wedges of lemon.

Shellfish and cephalopods Crab, prawns, oysters, mussels and squid are also abundant in most beachside locations.

Salads As for your lunchtime menus, salads will be in abundance, so ask for one to be served with your fish.

Foods to avoid

Too much bread Don't eat the entire breadbasket, or you'll not only be too full to enjoy your dinner but you will also be taking in extra calories that will make you feel bloated.

Crumbed, battered and fried fish can be deceiving Yes, the fish is healthy, but the outer layer isn't. Opt for grilled or steamed instead.

White rice or potatoes Many meals are served with them so avoid and request a salad or more vegetables instead.

Waterworks

On the journey

We all know that we should drink water when we fly, but how much is enough? You'll need one glass of water for every 30 minutes of flying. And remember that for every glass of alcohol you'll need to drink another glass of water to counteract the dehydrating effects. Let's hope the queue to the loo isn't too long!

When you're there

Remember that if it's hotter than usual you'll need to increase your liquid intake – around 2 litres of water is ideal, but drink more than that if it's immensely hot, or you've been drinking alcohol.

To drink or not to drink

Alcohol tends to play a large part in our holidays – nothing beats a glass of chilled white wine or a cocktail while the sun goes down. As for your food, drinking alcohol is all about moderation. Of course, you know all the health-and-safety reasons why you shouldn't get bladdered every night but you can still enjoy a few drinks. According to detox guru, Dr Joshi if you must drink, opt for vodka, as it's so purely distilled. Choose a health-giving mixer such as:

Cranberry – as every girl knows, it's good for cystitis
Pear – it's ideal if you're a bit blocked up
Mango – it's great for the skin
Orange – contains lots of vitamin C to keep your immune system high
Watermelon – there are practically no calories, but lots of hair-and-nail-strengthening vitamins
Pomegranate – it's packed with antioxidants, so you'll be partying all night long

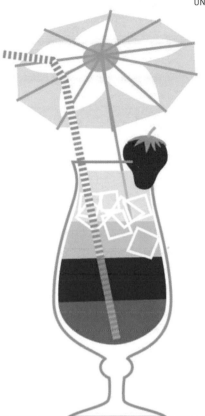

A Mars a day...

1 glass of white wine
Calories: 174
Equivalent to: just a little more than ²/₃ Mars Bar

1 vodka and tonic
Calories: 153
Equivalent to: ¹/₂ Mars Bar

1 gin and tonic
Calories: 150
Equivalent to: just under ¹/₂ Mars Bar

1 glass rosé
Calories: 170
Equivalent to:
²/₃ Mars Bar

1 glass of champagne
Calories: 80
Equivalent to:
¹/₃ Mars Bar

1 jug sangria
Calories 1,119
Equivalent to: 4 Mars Bars

1 glass of red wine
Calories: 160
Equivalent to:
²/₃ Mars Bar

1 pint lager
Calories: 163
Equivalent to:
1.7 Mars Bars

Health and fitness on holiday?

The following pages will help you find out how to make the most of your hotel facilities or environment to have a healthy holiday.

Make the most of your holiday

Lying beside the pool is a lovely way to spend your holiday, but, let's face it, it's not going to tone up those thighs. Try to do at least 1 hour of exercise each day. When it's sunny it's much easier to be active, without even realising you're doing so.

Toning activities

Sightseeing tones calves and, if you tighten your tummy muscles, you'll be strengthening your core muscles too.
Water volleyball is great for an all-over workout, including your arms, stomach and inner thighs.
Walking along the beach Walking along soft sand will challenge your calf muscles and tighten your inner thighs.
Swimming Aim to do about 20 lengths at a time in the pool for an all-over body workout. Beach volleyball will get your heart rate going.

Exercise	Calories burned	Drink equivalent
30 minutes' swimming	300	1 pina colada
30 minutes' frisbee	240	3 ½ glasses of vodka and soda
30 minutes' cycling	360	4 white wine spritzers
30 minutes' snorkelling	180	3 rum and diet colas
30 minutes' dancing	345	1 Long Island white tea

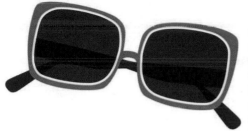

You gotta wear shades

Sunglasses not only protect your eyes from the sun and help you check out the lifeguard without being noticed, but they are also important to help protect your retinas from sun damage and UV rays. Here are some pointers to help when you're choosing:

- Black/polarised lenses reduce glare without distorting colours. They are also ideal if your head is suffering from the night before.
- Green/silver lenses enhance colour contrast so that colours remain true.
- Yellow/gold/purple/rose lenses filter out blue light caused by overcast weather. This means that colours appear more clearly, and you won't need to squint when you have sunny and cloudy conditions at the same time.
- Clear lenses are best kept for when it's very cloudy; wear sunglasses when outdoors at all other times.
- Make sure that the sunglasses fit and don't slide down your face when you bend down.
- If you wear spectacles, enquire about having prescription sunglasses as well.

Which sun factor should I use?

We all know how important it is to slip, slop and slap (suncream, that is). But despite this, more and more women are sunning themselves without using a sunblock or give a moment's thought to the damage they are doing to their skin, and health. Sunblock should be an everyday part of your beauty routine, even when it's cloudy, and most moisturisers now contain an SPF. But when you're on holiday a specific sunblock is necessary. Remember that a suntan might look healthy, but it's actually your skin's way of saying, 'Help, I'm damaged!' So, reduce the amount of damage to your skin by using at least a sun protection factor of 15, although most beauty experts recommend using no less than a 30 SPF on the face and a 15 on your body.

Do

- Apply sunscreen every hour – even water-resistant sunscreen should be reapplied. If you haven't been in the water, your body will still have sweated in the heat, thus reducing the effectiveness of the cream.
- Avoid the sun when it's at it's hottest between 11.00 am and 3.00 pm. Sit under an umbrella instead, or go sightseeing – but don't forget your wide-brimmed hat!
- Drink plenty of water to keep your skin from drying out.

Don't

- Forget to apply sunscreen to your ears, lips, nose, hands and feet.
- Ever go swimming without sunscreen on – the water increases the intensity of the sun's rays and you'll get even more burnt.
- Think that last year's sunscreen will still be effective. Buy a new tube for each holiday.
- Leave your sunscreen in the sun. Like you, it can be damaged by the sun's rays. Keep sunscreen well-covered and stored in the fridge at night.
- Ever use sunbeds. Cancer Research UK warns that 4 minutes of artificial tanning can cause as much damage as 1 hour in the midday sun

Get **beach-body** ready

If you've followed the beauty programme for your shape, you should be feeling smooth and tanned. If not, it's never too late to get your body bikini-ready. This quick-fix guide will help you.

Beauty problem
Dry hands
Solution

Your hands are the first area of your body to show signs of ageing, usually because we forget to moisturise them or apply sunblock. For a quick beauty fix, apply a good handful of intensive moisturising handcream and pop some socks on overnight or use cotton gloves if you have them. Leave for at least hours.

Beauty problem
Dry, cracked heels
Solution

Holidays, although good for the soul, are hell on your heels. All that sightseeing and salty water doesn't do your feet any favours. Apply a deep foot-conditioning moisturiser and wear socks to bed. If this isn't practical, when you're on the beach grab a handful of wet sand and scrub away at your heels. Remember to apply suncream to your feet as well as the rest of your body, so that they're moisturised throughout the day.

Beauty problem
Straggly bikini line
Solution

If you're exposing more than you mean to along your bikini line, it's time to get waxing or shaving. If it's the last minute and you don't have time to book an appointment, shave your legs, underarms and bikini line. Use an aloe vera oil (a baby oil with aloe vera is ideal) to avoid any ingrown and infected hair follicles. Many shavers now have built-in moisturising strips. Apply a deep, oil-based moisturiser after shaving while your skin is still damp. This will lock in the moisture and give you seriously smooth, buff legs.

Beauty problem
Streaky self-tanner
Solution

Even the most expertly applied self-tanner can become streaky and blotchy. If this has happened to you, don't panic! Instead, using an exfoliator or facecloth, rub at the area to loosen the tanning product. Then apply some lemon juice to the area to encourage the tanning pigmentation to fade a little. If the self-tanner you've bought

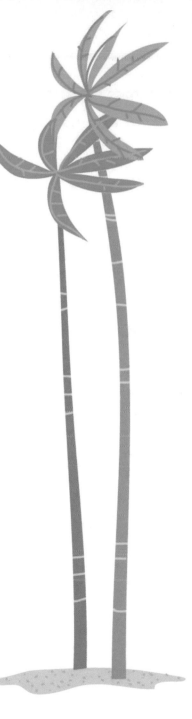

is too dark for your skin tone, mix one dollop of fake tan with two dollops of body moisturiser. This will give you a lighter tan and streaks will be less visible.

How to look like a model in your holiday snaps

If you're one of the 2.5 million sufferers from a bad back, then correcting your posture will simultaneously alleviate back pain and make you instantly appear 5lb slimmer. 'Round shoulders make your stomach sag and add the illusion of excess weight,' says Pilates expert Lynne Robinson. 'Imagine that there is a balloon attached to your head, and try to create as much space as possible between your jaw and your shoulders. You'll immediately look slimmer.'

Try a daily Pilates workout to strengthen and flatten your stomach. Draw up your pelvic floor muscles and lower your stomach backwards towards your spine, exhaling on release. Repeat as often as you can throughout the day: on the sun lounger, lilo or your beach towel.

Be photogenic

If you run to hide behind the closest palm tree whenever somebody attempts to take a picture of you in your bikini, you're probably missing out on some great holiday snaps. Make your thighs look slimmer and define your waistline by angling your hips 45° away from the camera. Bend your front knee slightly. Angle your shoulders towards the camera, pull your shoulders back to create an illusion of height, and rest your hands on your hips. Your arms will help draw attention away from your waist. Above all, smile! There's nothing more attractive than a happy, confident person. You're on holiday remember!

Recipes

Apple, Vegetable and Quorn Curry

Put 2 tsp **curry paste**, 1 tsp **chutney**, 3 sliced **tomatoes**, 1 tbsp **sultanas**, 1 tbsp water in a pan. Cook for 2 minutes. Add ¼ pack **Quorn** and ½ sliced onion. Simmer 5 minutes. Add ½ sliced **pepper** and 1 small chopped **carrot**. Cook for 5 minutes (add more water if necessary). Add 4 sliced **mushrooms** and cook for 1 minute. Just before serving, add ½ sliced **celery** stick and ¼ sliced **apple**. Heat through.

Baked Spicy Chicken and Rice

Preheat the oven to 190°C/375°F/Gas 5. Heat ½ tbsp olive oil in a frying pan. Add 2 **chicken** thighs, fry over a high heat until golden brown. Remove and set aside. Add ½ chopped **onion** to the pan; sweat gently for 6 minutes. Stir in 1 crushed **garlic** clove, ½ tsp **garam masala**, ¼ tsp ground **ginger**, ¼ sliced **green chilli**. Stir in 75g **brown basmati rice** and cook for 1 minute. Pour into a small ovenproof dish. Top with the chicken and pour over 160ml hot **chicken stock**. Cover with foil and bake for 20 minutes, or until the rice has absorbed the stock. Add hot water if necessary. Uncover and stir in 50g frozen **mixed green vegetables**. Re-cover and bake for 10 more minutes.

Beef Fajitas

Preheat the grill to medium-high. Rub 100g lean **beef** with 1 tsp **sunflower oil** and sprinkle with 1 tsp **fajita seasoning**. Grill 4 minutes on each side. Rest the beef for 5 minutes. Slice thinly then divide between 2 warmed **flour tortillas** and add ½ each **red and green pepper**, sliced, and 1 small, sliced **red onion**. Roll up and serve.

Beetroot, Parsley and Feta Salad

Steam 350g raw **beetroot** for 40 minutes, or until tender, peel. Cool. Fry 3 chopped **shallots** and ½ chopped **red chilli** in ½ tbsp oil. Cut beetroot into wedges and add ¼ tbsp **cumin seeds**, 2 tbsp chopped fresh **parsley** and 75g crumbled **feta** cheese. Season with **black pepper**.

Broccoli Blowout

Put 435g fresh **broccoli** florets into a steamer and add 140g **green beans** and 1 **carrot**, sliced into strips. Steam until almost tender, then add a handful of fresh **spinach**. Meanwhile, cook 150g **chicken**, **turkey** or **fish** in a pan with a little stock or milk. Season with **pepper** then serve on a bed of the steamed vegetables.

Carrot and Coriander Soup

Heat 1 tsp **olive oil** in a pan and cook ½ **onion** until tender. Add 125g **carrots**, chopped, and cook for 5–10 minutes until soft. Stir in 1 medium chopped **potato**, 1 tsp ground **coriander** and season with **pepper**. Add 400ml vegetable stock. Simmer until the vegetables are tender. Blend and serve with chopped fresh **coriander**.

Chicken Salad

Grill 1 small skinless **chicken** breast with 1 tsp oil. Put ½ **avocado** in a bowl with 2 quartered **tomatoes** and the torn leaves of ¼ head of **lettuce**. When the chicken is ready, leave to cool. Toast a handful of **pine nuts** in a small pan over medium heat to lightly brown. Slice the chicken and add to the salad. Sprinkle with **pine nuts**. Add **lemon juice** and **pepper**.

Cottage Pie

Dry-fry 115g extra-lean minced **beef** until brown. Add 1 chopped small **onion** and 1 crushed **garlic** clove. Fry until soft. Stir in 150ml **beef stock**, 1 tbsp **tomato purée** and 1 tsp **Worcestershire sauce**. Boil, cover and simmer until the gravy has thickened. Boil 1 large peeled **potato** and mash with 1 tbsp **skimmed milk**. Put the mince in an ovenproof dish. Top with the mash and 1 tbsp grated reduced-fat **Cheddar** cheese. Grill until the cheese melts.

Dairy-free Cream of Broccoli Soup

Gently fry 1 small sliced **leek** in ½ tbsp **sunflower oil** with 1 chopped **garlic** clove and 1 **bay leaf** until the leek is soft. Add 120g **broccoli** and 150ml **vegetable stock**. Boil, then cover and simmer for 10 minutes. Remove the bay leaf and blend the soup. Return to the pan. Add a few drops of **lemon juice**, **pepper** and 3 tbsp **dairy-free soya cream**. Heat through.

Energy Smoothie

Blend 1 **banana**, 150ml **low-fat soya milk**, 1 tsp **honey**, 1 tbsp mixed **sunflower and pumpkin seeds**, a little freshly grated **nutmeg**.

Feta and Roasted Tomato Pasta Salad

Preheat the oven to 220°C/425°F/Gas 7. Put 50g **feta** cheese in a piece of foil, drizzle with a little **oil** and wrap into a parcel. Place at one end of a shallow ovenproof dish. Pour 1 tbsp oil into the dish and add 10 **cherry tomatoes** or 3 **vine tomatoes**. Bake for 15 minutes or until the tomatoes are soft. Meanwhile, cook 50g wheat-free or **wholemeal pasta** according to the pack instructions. Remove the tomatoes and cheese from the oven. Combine with the pasta. Add 50g **black olives**, 15g **pine nuts** and a handful of **basil leaves**, if you like.

Fish in Sleeping Bags

Preheat the oven to 180°C/350°F/Gas 4. Put a piece of foil on a baking tray and lay 1 small **cod** fillet on top. Put 1 sliced **tomato**, ½ sliced **onion**, ½ sliced **green pepper**, ½ diced **courgette** and 4 sliced **mushrooms** over the top. Season with pepper and fold up the foil to make a parcel. Bake for 25–30 minutes, or until cooked through. Meanwhile, cook ½ cup **brown basmati rice** according to the pack instructions. Serve the fish on the rice.

Fish Pie

Preheat the oven to 190°C/375°F/Gas 5. Boil 125g floury **potatoes** and 150g **swede**, in chunks. Put 50g low-fat **soft cheese** with **garlic** and herbs into a pan with 3 tbsp **vegetable stock**. Heat slowly, blending until smooth. Blend 1 tsp **cornflour** with 1 tbsp cold water and stir into the cheese mixture. Add 150g skinless, boneless **cod**, cut into large dice, and 1 tsp chopped fresh **parsley**. Stir, then pour into a small ovenproof dish. Drain and mash the swede and potato. Spoon over the fish. Bake for 25 minutes, or until browned.

Five-spice Chicken Stir-fry

Heat 1 tsp sunflower oil in a wok and stir-fry 1 small sliced skinless **chicken** breast. Add 1 small bag ready-prepared **stir-fry vegetables** and 1 tsp **Chinese five-spice** powder. Stir-fry until the vegetables are cooked but still crisp. Season with a dash of reduced-salt soy sauce.

Garlic Mushroom Spaghetti

Heat 1 tsp **olive oil** and fry 65g **chestnut mushrooms** over a high heat for 3 minutes. Reduce the heat and add ½ crushed **garlic** clove. Fry for 1 minute, then tip into a bowl with 1 tbsp chopped fresh **parsley**. Heat 2 tsp oil in another pan and fry ½ chopped small **onion** and 1 chopped **celery** stick for 5 minutes. Stir in 100g canned chopped **tomatoes** and ¼ chopped **red chilli**. Boil and simmer uncovered for 10 minutes. Meanwhile cook the **spaghetti** and drain. Toss with the sauce and top with the mushrooms.

Ginger and Garlic Beef

Heat ½ tbsp **sunflower oil** in a wok. Add 100g **beef**, thinly sliced in strips, and brown quickly. Add 1 tsp grated fresh **root ginger**, 1 crushed **garlic** clove and 2 chopped **spring onions**. Cook for 2 minutes. Add ½ tbsp **soy sauce**. Steam ½ head of **pak choi**, sliced, and 25g **mangetouts** until tender. Toss with **sesame oil**. Serve with the beef.

Grape Shakes

Juice 3–4 **oranges**, peeled, 1 **kiwi fruit** and 1 **apple**. Pour into a blender and add a handful of **grapes**, 1 tsp **honey** and 1 tbsp **sunflower seeds** (optional). (Grapes contain fantastic detoxifying ingredients, so this is an ideal way to continue with your healthy-eating plan and eliminate any bloating.)

Lamb with Aubergine and Raisins

Preheat the oven to 180°C/350°F/Gas 4. Put 1 tbsp **olive oil** into an ovenproof dish and add 40g diced **lamb**, ½ diced **aubergine**, ½ diced **sweet potato**, 6 mushrooms and 1 tbsp **raisins**. Toss with the oil. Pour about 75ml **vegetable stock** over the lamb to cover and bake for 40–60 minutes, or until tender. Serve over **couscous**.

Lemon-drizzled Fish

Put 1 tbsp finely grated lemon rind in a bowl and combine with 2 tbsp chopped fresh **parsley** and seasoning. Press onto both sides of 1 fillet of **white fish** (such as cod or haddock). Heat 1 tbsp **olive oil** in a frying pan and fry the fish until cooked through. Serve with **lemon wedges** and steamed **vegetables**.

Lime, Tomato and Scallop Salad

Put 50g dried **rice noodles** in a bowl, cover with boiling water, and soak until just tender. Drain and rinse under cold water. Combine 1 tsp **sweet chilli sauce** and 1 tsp **lime juice** in a bowl. Grill 150g **white scallops**, brushing with the chilli mixture, until cooked. Steam 75g chopped **asparagus**, until just tender. Rinse under cold water and drain. Make a dressing: mix 1 tbsp **peanut oil**, a pinch of **brown sugar**, ¼ tbsp each chopped fresh **coriander** and **mint** leaves, ¼ small, chopped **red chilli** and 15ml **lime juice**. Toss the noodles, scallops and asparagus in a large bowl with 75g halved **yellow tomatoes** and the dressing. Sprinkle with 15g toasted flaked **almonds**.

Marinated Chicken with Prune Salsa

Mix 1 tbsp **olive oil**, 1 tsp **tomato purée**, 1 tsp **honey** and 1 tsp **soy sauce**. Spread over 1 small skinless chicken **breast**. Marinate for 1 hour, turning halfway through. Make a salsa: put 50g ready-to-eat **prunes** in a pan with a little water and bring to the boil. Leave to soak for 10 minutes. In a bowl, combine ½ chopped **chilli**, 1 chopped medium **tomato**, 1 tsp **olive oil** and juice of ½ **lime**. Chop the prunes, then add to the salsa. Chill. Grill the chicken for 15 minutes or until cooked through. Add 1 tbsp each of **coriander** and **mint** to the salsa.

Mediterranean Roasted Vegetable Soup

Preheat the oven to 200°C/400°F/Gas 6. Heat 1 tbsp **olive oil** in a roasting tin in the oven for 3 minutes. Add 1 sliced **courgette**, ½ diced **aubergine**, ¼ each chopped **red and yellow pepper**, 1 sliced **garlic** clove, 1 tsp **rosemary** leaves, and seasoning. Turn to coat, then bake for 20 minutes, stirring occasionally. Add 1 packet vine **tomatoes** and stir to coat. Bake for 25 minutes. Boil 150ml vegetable stock in a pan. Blend the roasted **vegetables**, add the stock and whiz until almost smooth. Pour back into the pan and reheat, stirring. Spoon into a bowl and top with 1 tbsp **pesto**, 1 tbsp **crème fraîche** or **soya cream**, and a few **basil** leaves.

Millet Lunch

Put 50g **millet** in a large bowl and pour over just enough boiling water to cover. Leave it to stand for 45 minutes until the liquid is absorbed and the **millet** is cool. Use a fork to break into fine grains. Stir in ¼ diced **red** onion, ½ diced **avocado**, ¼ diced **red pepper**, 2 **cherry tomatoes**, quartered; 20g **mushrooms**. (The vegetables should be raw, but you can lightly steam them first, if you prefer). Whisk together 1½ tbsp **olive oil**, ½ tbsp **cider vinega**r, 1 tbsp chopped fresh **mixed herbs**, 1 tsp **tahini paste**, 1 tsp **lemon juice**, **sea salt** and **black pepper**. Toss through the **salad** with 1 tbsp mixed **pumpkin** and **sunflower seeds**.

Minestrone Soup

Fry 1 chopped **onion** in ½ tbsp **oil** for 5 minutes, or until softened. Add 2 crushed **garlic cloves** and 100g diced **ham** or **pancetta**. Add 400g can chopped **tomatoes** and 400g can mixed **beans**. Cook for 2 minutes, then add 900ml hot **vegetable stock**. Add ¼ cup small wheat-free pasta shapes. Simmer for 20 minutes. Serve a bowl and freeze any remaining for another day.

Moroccan Lamb

Dry-fry 150g **lamb neck** fillet in a non-stick frying pan. Add 2 tsp **paprika** and 3 tsp ground **cinnamon**, and fry for 1 minute. Add 400g can chopped **tomatoes** and 1 tbsp chopped fresh **parsley**. Bring to the boil, then cover and simmer 30 minutes, or until the **lamb** is tender.

Muesli

Mix together ¼ cup each of oat flakes, **millet flakes** and **brown rice flakes** with dried **apricots, peaches** and **cranberries**. Soak in **soya** or **rice milk** overnight or 1 hour before breakfast. Add 1 tbsp ground **mixed seeds and nuts** such as **almonds, hazelnuts, pecan nuts, walnuts** and **Brazil nuts**. Top with live, **natural yogurt**.

New You Boot Camp Smoothie.

Whiz together 250g **blueberries**, 250g **raspberries**, 100g **oats**, 1 tsp **seeds**, 200ml **apple juice**, 6 tsp **organic honey** (preferably manuka), 600ml **soya yogurt** in a food processor or blender. Drink immediately.

Noodle Salad with Chilli Lemongrass Dressing

Put the following in a screwtop jar: 1 tbsp **olive oil**, 1 tsp **sesame oil**, juice of ½ **lime**, 1 tsp chopped fresh **coriander**, ½ **red chilli**, seeded and chopped, 1cm fresh **lemongrass**, chopped, ½ tsp **honey**. Shake to mix. Cook 100g fresh **egg noodles** according to the pack instructions. Drain and rinse under cold water. Put into a bowl, and add 1 **carrot**, cut into ribbons, ½ sliced **pak choi**, 20g halved **mangetouts**, 1 tsp **sesame seeds**. Toss with the dressing.

Nutty Fruit Shake

In a blender whiz 200ml **semi-skimmed milk** (or dairy-free alternative) with 1 tbsp **wheatgerm**, 100g fresh or frozen **raspberries**, 2 tsp **honey**, a handful of **seeds**.

Paprika Pork

Heat ¼ tbsp **olive oil** in a pan and add 1 **onion**, thinly sliced. Fry over a low-medium heat, stirring occasionally, for 10–15 minutes, or until soft and lightly coloured. Add 150g **pork** fillet, cut into bite-size chunks, and stir over high heat to seal and brown. Stir in ½ tbsp **paprika**. Cook briefly, then add 75ml **chicken stock** and bring to the boil. Cover and simmer for 30–35 minutes, or until the **pork** is tender. Stir in 50ml **low-fat crème fraîche** and simmer for 2 minutes.

Pea and Broad Bean Soup

Put 60g frozen **peas** into a pan with 60g frozen **broad beans** and 225ml **vegetable stock**. Boil, cover and simmer for 30 minutes, or until tender. Season and blend until smooth.

Pomegranate Lentil Soup

Melt ½ tbsp **butter or margarine** in a large pan and cook ½ chopped medium **onion** over low-medium heat until tender. Add 300ml water, 25g **lentils**, 30g long-grain **brown rice**, ¼ tsp **turmeric** and **seasoning**. Bring to the boil, then reduce the heat and cover. Simmer over a low heat for 40 minutes or until the **lentils** and **rice** are tender. Add 1 tbsp chopped fresh **parsley**, 3 chopped **spring onions** and 3 tbsp **pomegranate juice**. Simmer for 15 minutes. Melt ¼ tbsp **butter or margarine** in a small frying pan. Add ½ tbsp **fresh mint**. Cook gently until the **butter or margarine** is golden brown. Pour over the soup. Sprinkle with 1 tsp **raisins**.

Power Plate

Juice 1 **orange**, peeled; 250g **carrots**; 125g **beetroot**; 125g **strawberries** and blend if required. Drink immediately.

Power porridge

Put ½ cup rolled **oats**, 2 cups **water**, 1 cup chopped fresh or frozen **fruit** (try berries, peaches, melons, apples), 1 tsp **cinnamon** and 1 tsp **vanill**a in a microwave-safe bowl. Cover (leaving one side vented) and microwave for 2 minutes. Stir and microwave for a further 1–2 minutes. Add a little manuka **honey**.

Prawn and Vegetable Skewers

Lightly grill or fry 150g fresh **prawns** to ensure they're evenly cooked through. Preheat the grill. Thread the **prawns** onto **skewers**, alternating with the following ingredients: ½ **pepper**, cut into large chunks, 1 large **onion**, quartered, 100g **mushrooms**, quartered, 100g **pineapple** chunks (fresh or canned), 50g **courgette**, cut into thick slices. Brush with a little **honey or olive oil**, if you like. Put on a baking tray and grill, turning, for 4–5 minutes, or until cooked through. Serve the **skewers** with a **green salad**.

Rice Jumble

Put ¼ each **red, green and yellow pepper** on a grill rack, skin-side uppermost. Grill for 10 minutes, or until skin is charred. Place in a plastic bag, seal and leave for 5 minutes or until the skins have loosened, then peel the skins and slice thinly. Cook 75g **long grain brown rice** in a pan of boiling water for 25–30 minutes, or until tender. Drain, refresh under cold water and drain again. Mix the **rice and peppers** in a large bowl with 1 diced **vine tomato**, ½ **grated medium courgette** and 1 tbsp torn **basil** leaves. Make a dressing: 2 tsp **olive oil**, ½ crushed **garlic** clove, 1 tsp **honey**, ¼ tsp maple **syrup and black pepper**. Drizzle over the **salad**.

Soya Bean Salad

Steam 2 cups frozen **soya beans** for 5 minutes, or until crisp-tender. Drain, rinse with cold water and drain again. In a large bowl, mix the **beans** with 2 sliced **spring onions**, 2 seeded and diced **tomatoes** and 1 tbsp chopped fresh **basil**. Make a dressing: mix together 1 tbsp fresh **lime juice**, 1 tsp honey, 1 tsp **Dijon mustard**, 2 tsp **olive oil**. Toss with the **vegetables** and season with **black pepper**.

Spinach Salad with Garlic Dressing

Put 1 large handful baby **spinach** leaves and 3 **sun-dried tomatoes** or 6 **cherry tomatoes** in a bowl. (If you prefer, you can heat this up briefly in a frying pan with a little **olive oil**.) Put 1 tbsp **olive oil** in a pan and add 1 sliced **garlic** clove, ½ tbsp rinsed salted **capers**, 1 tbsp **olives**, ½ tbsp **lemon juice**, ½ tbsp fresh **thyme leaves** and **black pepper**. Heat for 1 minute, then pour some over the **vegetables**.

Strawberry Starter Smoothie

Blend 5 **strawberries**, hulled, a handful of **blueberries**, a handful of **raspberries**, 1 **banana**, 1 tbsp **dairy-free yogurt**, a handful of mixed **pumpkin** and **sunflower seeds**, 300ml **apple juice**.

Stuffed Potato Boats

Boil 1 egg-sized **potato** in its skin for 20–25 minutes, or until tender. Cut in half and scoop out the inside. Mash with a fork. Gently fry ½ **onion** and ½ chopped **garlic glove** in 1 tsp **olive oil** until soft. Mix the **onion** with 25g chopped **cashew nuts**, 1 tbsp **breadcrumbs**, a pinch of **mixed herbs** and **seasoning**. Mix with the **potato**, add ½ beaten **egg** and mix well. Brush the **potato** skins with a little **oil**, heap the mixture into the halves, and bake for 10–15 minutes, or until golden.

Super-sporty Stir-fry

Slice into strips 4–6 **shiitake mushrooms**, 1 **green pepper**, 1 **carrot**, 6 **mangetouts**, ½ **courgette** and 1 **pak choi**. Heat ½ tbsp **oil** in a wok or pan, then cook all the **vegetables** except the **pak choi**. Meanwhile cook ½ cup brown basmati rice, or a small portion of glass noodles, according to the directions on the pack. When the stir-fry is almost cooked, add the pak choi and cook until the leaves are limp.

Thai Green Curry with Prawns

Heat 1 tbsp oil in a wok or large pan. Add ½ chopped onion and cook for 3 minutes, or until soft. Add ½ can low-fat coconut milk and bring to the boil. Lower the heat and add ½−1 tbsp Thai green curry paste, according to taste. Stir and simmer for 5 minutes. Add ½ sliced courgette, 4 sliced shiitake mushrooms, 15g mangetouts, 15g baby corn and 7 uncooked king prawns. Cook for 5 minutes or until the prawns are pink and the vegetables are tender.

Thai Salmon

Heat the grill to high. Place 1 small salmon fillet in a shallow ovenproof dish and grill for 5 minutes, or until just cooked through. Cover and set aside. Heat a wok with ½ tsp sunflower oil and add ½ tsp grated fresh root ginger, ¼ sliced mild red chilli and 3 sliced spring onions. Stir-fry for 2−3 minutes. Stir in 1 tsp soy sauce, a pinch of sugar and a splash of water, then take off the heat. Add 1 tbsp chopped fresh coriander to the chilli mixture and serve with the salmon.

Three-bean Salad

Drain and rinse ½ can mixed beans, and mix with ½ chopped onion, 2 finely chopped celery sticks, ¼ chopped cucumber, 2 diced tomatoes and a little chopped red chilli, to taste. Add lemon juice and black pepper.

Tomato Soup

Heat 1 tbsp olive oil in a large pan and cook ½ chopped onion for 5 minutes, or until soft. Add 1 chopped carrot, 2 peeled and chopped potatoes, 2 chopped large organic tomatoes, and 400g can tomatoes. Bring to the boil then simmer for 30 minutes, or until the vegetables are tender. Add 1 tbsp chopped basil and black pepper to taste.

Tuna and Sweetcorn Pesto Pasta

Cook 50g wholewheat pasta and lightly steam 5 broccoli florets. Toss together, with 1 tbsp pesto, 1 chopped tomato, 2 tbsp steamed sweetcorn, ½ small can tuna in brine. Sprinkle with 1 tbsp grated Parmesan cheese.

Tuna Meatballs

Flake 80g canned tuna into a bowl and add 1 tbsp pine nuts, the grated zest of ¼ lemon and 2 tbsp chopped fresh parsley. Mix with 15g fresh breadcrumbs, ¼ beaten egg and seasoning until completely combined. Roll into small balls. Cook 30g wholemeal spaghetti. Heat ½ tbsp olive oil in a large non-stick frying pan and fry the tuna balls for 5 minutes, turning every minute until golden. Drain on kitchen paper. Heat 100g tomato pasta sauce (from a jar or home-made) and toss together with the pasta and tuna balls.

Vegetable Fajitas

Heat the oven to 180°C/350°F/Gas 4. Wrap 2 wholemeal fajitas in foil and warm in the oven for 10 minutes. Heat 1 tbsp olive oil in a pan and cook ½ chopped onion until soft. Add 3−4 cauliflower florets and Cook for 5 minutes. Put 150g chickpeas, drained and rinsed, in another pan with 150g arrabiata

sauce. Simmer for 2–3 minutes. Add 1 tbsp
fresh chopped **coriander**. Put this **sauce**
into a small bowl. Put 75g **low-fat yogurt** and
15g **baby spinach** into bowls and use all to
fill the **fajitas**.

Vegetarian Flan

Preheat the oven to 200°C/400°F/Gas 6. Toss
½ thickly sliced **courgette**, ¼ sliced red
pepper and ½ sliced **red onion** in 1 tbsp **olive
oil**. Put in a roasting tin and roast for
30 minutes. Take the vegetables from oven.
Add 25g **sun-dried tomatoes**. Stir and cool.
Reduce oven to 190°C/375°F/Gas 5. Roll out
65g ready-made **wholemeal pastry** and line
a 10cm individual flan tin or popover tin.
Spread 1 tsp **Dijon mustard** over the pastry
and sprinkle over 25g grated **Gruyère cheese**,
with the **vegetables** on top. Beat 1 egg with
30ml **Alpro dairy-free soya milk** and ½ tbsp
chopped fresh **chives**, then pour over the
vegetables. Bake for 20–25 minutes, or until
set and golden.

Vietnamese Chicken Noodle Soup

Put 300ml **chicken stock** into a pan with
5mm peeled fresh **root ginger**, ½ star anise,
¼ **cinnamon stick**, 1 tbsp **fish sauce**, and
½ skinless **chicken breast**. Slowly bring to
the boil, reduce the heat and poach for 8
minutes. Remove the **chicken** and leave to
rest for 5 minutes, then shred. Soak 50g wide
rice noodles according to the pack
instructions, then drain and put into a bowl.
Strain the stock into the bowl. Top with
shredded **chicken**, 25g **beansprouts**, 1 sliced
spring onion, a small handful each of fresh
coriander and **mint**, chopped, and serve
with a wedge of lime.

Vegetarians

If you're a vegetarian, or vegan, you
can still use the recipes in this
book, but you will need to adapt
them slightly. The meat and fish
recipes can work with vegetarian
substitutes, such as tofu, tempeh,
soya protein and Quorn, or add
1/3 can of beans or a small handful
of nuts. Remember that as a
vegetarian you are prone to low
blood sugar levels and anaemia, so
make sure you eat enough protein
– even if it's just a handful of nuts
or a small tub of low-fat yogurt –
and boost your iron levels by eating
plenty of leafy greens.

Cook more!

····➤ Each recipe serves one
person, but you can easily
double up the quantities to
serve two, or multiply them
to serve more people.
····➤ As they're tasty and
nutritious, they make great
meals even when you've
finished the diet plan. Enjoy!

Index